the total
DESTRESS PLAN

For Denis, Always

THIS IS A CARLTON BOOK

Text copyright © 2002 Beth MacEoin
Design and special photography copyright
© 2002 Carlton Books Limited

First published in 2002.
This edition published in 2011
by Carlton Books Limited
20 Mortimer Street
London W1T 3JW

10 9 8 7 6 5 4 3 2 1

A CIP catalogue record for this book
is available from the British Library

ISBN 978 1 84732 555 6

Printed and bound in China.

The author and publisher have made
every effort to ensure that all information
is correct and up to date at the time of
publication. Neither the author nor the
publisher can accept responsibility for
any accident, injury or damage that
results from using the ideas, information
or advice offered in this book.

The application and quality of beauty
products, beauty treatments, herbal
preparations and essential oils is beyond
the control of the above parties, who
cannot be held responsible for any
problems resulting from their use. Always
follow the manufacturer's instructions
and if in doubt, seek further advice.

Do not use herbal preparations or
essential oils without prior consultation
with a qualified practitioner or medical
doctor if you are pregnant, taking any
form of medication, or if you suffer
from oversensitive skin.

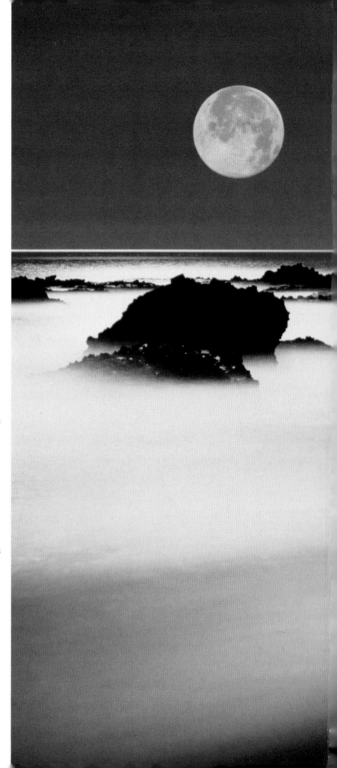

the total
DESTRESS
PLAN

a lifestyle action plan for reducing
anxiety and enhancing relaxation

Beth MacEoin

CARLTON
BOOKS

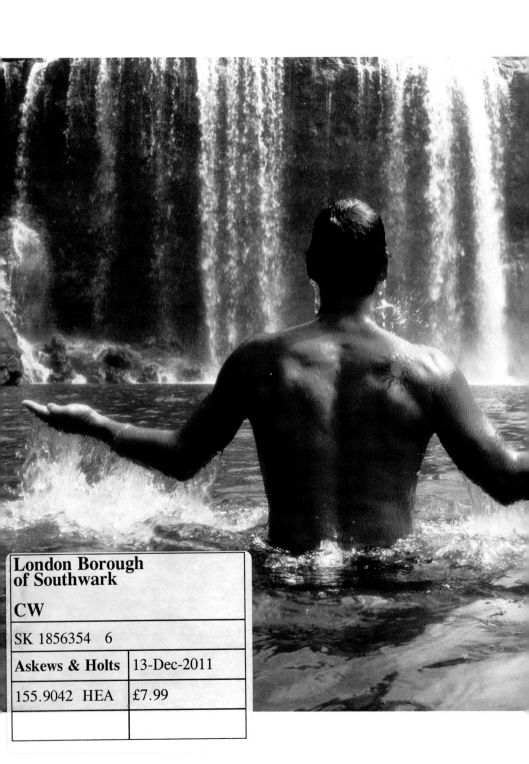

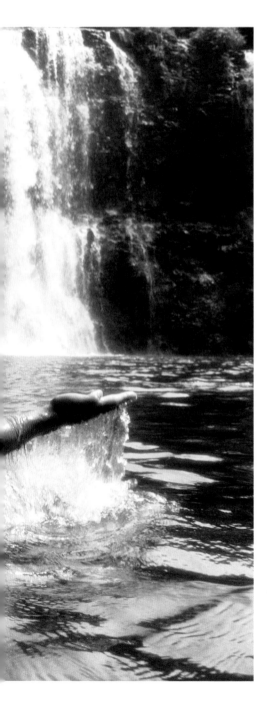

contents

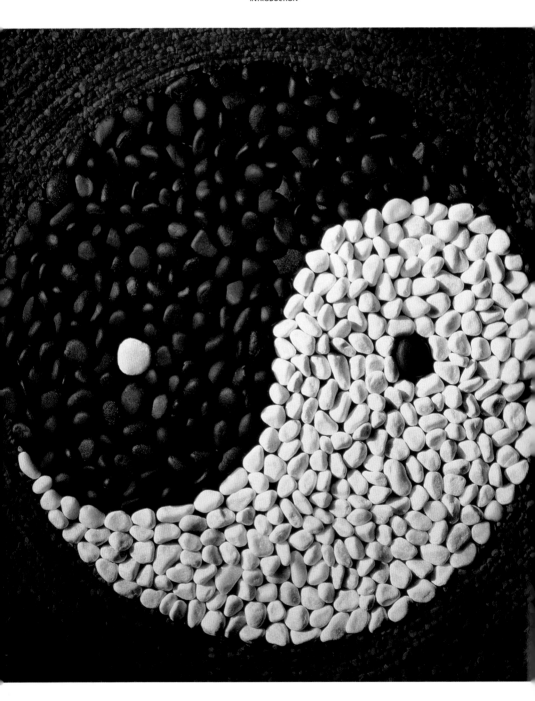

Introduction

Stress is all around us: it is how we handle it that counts. Whether we interpret feeling stressed as a positive or a negative influence depends on many complex factors – from our mental and emotional make-up to the quality of our professional lives. Everyone is likely to have a strong opinion about stress: there are those who believe that complaining about it is strictly for the feeble, and those who are adamant that it is one of the most negative aspects of twenty-first-century living. The one thing about stress that is undeniably true is that we cannot ignore it.

Stress is here to stay, so it makes good sense to explore practical ways to tame it and turn it to our advantage. By harnessing the creative fallout of stress, we can use it to fuel activities that require us to be fired up and at our sharpest mentally. By identifying and using practical tools for stress management and relaxation we can also make sure that we fully unwind.

left THE YIN-YANG SYMBOL DENOTES THE OPTIMUM STATE OF BALANCE THAT WE AIM TO ACHIEVE IN OUR LIFESTYLE.

By consciously creating this essential balance in our lives, we are likely to find that we experience a new sense of being masters and mistresses of our stress levels rather than slaves to them. Once we assume the controls with regard to effective stress management, we will be delighted to find ourselves more emotionally stable, increasingly sharp and productive mentally, and in better physical shape, too. This is because the way we respond to stress has a profound effect on all aspects of our experience. Thus any successful approach to stress management has to be generated from a holistic perspective.

Making Stress-Busting Techniques Work for Us

How this book should be used is up to each individual reading it: the chances are that no two readers are going to absorb identical benefits from it – and this is exactly as it should be. After all, one of the basic ideas common to all forms of complementary and alternative medicine is that each person's make-up is unique and that any medical advice needs to be finely tailored to fit this special combination of emotional and mental features. This is as true of this book as of any alternative medical consultation; it is the aim of the advice given in the following pages to provide each reader with a plan of action that will enable them to manage stress – whether it comes from a mental, emotional or physical direction (or an unfortunate combination of all three at once). If we apply the principles outlined in the following pages, we should also find that our overall health benefits immensely, as we are encouraged, gently but firmly, to make in the vulnerable areas of our lives those positive changes that we may have been putting off for a very long time.

Some of us may decide that we need a radical health-and-lifestyle overhaul because we feel constantly strung up or wrung out; we have problems sleeping; we suffer from a constant, low-grade headache; we never enjoy our food; or we seem to lurch from one minor infection to another. If this sounds familiar, do make a point of reading the whole book. By following the basic principles that make up the de-stress plan, it will be easier for you to put in place a sound, basic foundation that will not only help you to relax and unwind, but will also increase your energy levels, promote restful and refreshing sleep, and boost your inbuilt defences so that recurrent infections will gradually become a dim and distant memory.

Alternatively, those of us who have developed a framework for our lifestyle that is generally sound and balanced but feel that there is one area, such as exercise, nutrition or relaxation, that we know is less than perfect might choose to head straight for the relevant chapter in order to get to work as speedily as possible. Chapter Two will help you identify the nature and level of stress from which you are suffering.

The book has been structured to be as accessible and flexible as possible, so that each chapter can be read as a complete, self-contained section. Nevertheless, the text does, as a whole, follow a logical sequence: from a basic understanding of how unmanaged stress has a negative effect on our minds and emotions, we move to practical strategies for dealing with the physical problems that arise as a direct consequence of having to deal with too much stress for too long.

Before all this begins to sound like just too much hard work, it may reassure you to know that *The Total De-stress Plan* has been deliberately designed to avoid anything punishing, spartan or impossible to incorporate into a busy lifestyle. Moreover, there are plenty of luxurious treats included in the plan for those of us who enjoy a thorough pampering – as often as possible.

Most importantly, it is worth emphasizing that once we begin to experience the multiple benefits that flow from maintaining a more balanced lifestyle, we are likely to find that we want, and find it second nature, to stick to the basic principles of the de-stress plan. Whatever your reasons for reading this book, and whatever your aims, I wish you the best of health on your journey.

right **TO GAIN MAXIMUM BENEFIT FROM** *THE TOTAL DE-STRESS PLAN,* **TAKE TIME TO THINK ABOUT WHAT YOUR SPECIFIC INDIVIDUAL NEEDS ARE.**

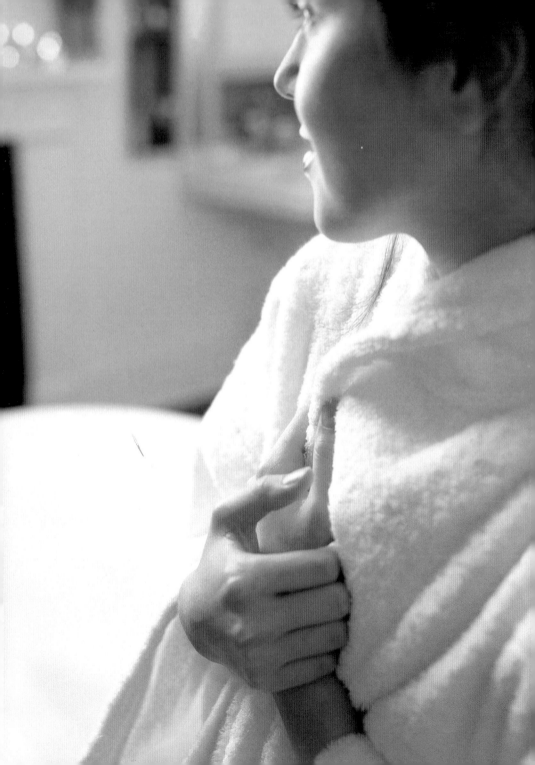

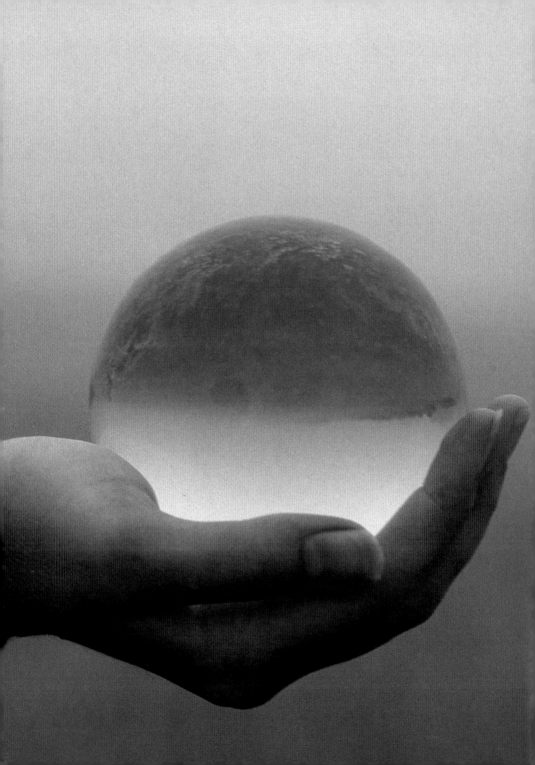

Good Versus Bad: The Double-Edged Nature of Stress

Stress: Friend or Foe?

IT IS TRUE TO SAY THAT ONE PERSON'S STRESS IS ANOTHER PERSON'S STIMULUS FOR ACTION. AS A RESULT, SOMETHING THAT MAY BE REGARDED WITH DREAD AND FEAR BY ONE PERSON MAY GIVE ANOTHER A REAL 'BUZZ', MAKING THEM FEEL MORE ALIVE, AND ENCOURAGING THEM TO PERFORM AT PEAK CAPACITY.

This is partly because of the way in which stress can manifest itself in a surprisingly wide range of guises: a tight deadline at work, speaking in public, having a heated argument with someone we are normally close to, developing a severe illness, moving house, experiencing financial pressure, having a baby, going through the break-up of a relationship, falling in love, going on holiday, or starting a new job.

Some of these items may surprise you. Indeed, the list includes some very exciting and pleasurable experiences, life events that we would expect to welcome – falling in love, for example, or moving on to a new situation at work that broadens our possibilities and raises our prospects. After all, we all know that stress is usually connected to events that are essentially negative in nature, don't we?

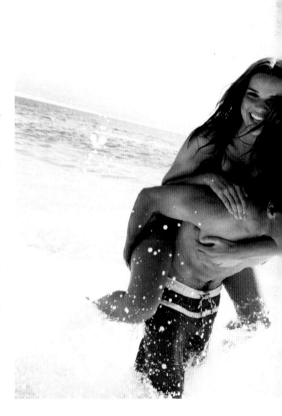

left A HAPPY AND HEALTHY LIFE DEPENDS ON ACHIEVING A BALANCE BETWEEN POSITIVE AND NEGATIVE STRESS.
right PLEASURE-FILLED AND CAREFREE EXPERIENCES CAN BE POWERFUL ALLIES IN THE BATTLE AGAINST NEGATIVE STRESS.

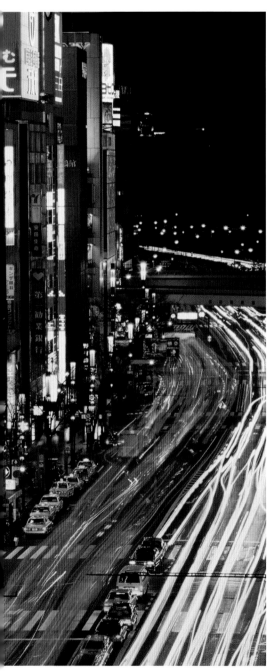

left **BEING CAUGHT UP IN TRAFFIC JAM CAN SEND NEGATIVE STRESS LEVELS SOARING.**

The reality of stress is rather more complex and fascinating, as we will discover. The stress response is activated when we are under pressure and required to adapt to an unfamiliar or changed situation: our capacity to manage stress will determine whether we interpret this situation as threatening or pleasurable. This, in turn, will depend strongly on our ability to adapt to and welcome changing circumstances. What we need to do, therefore, is build up our emotional, mental and physical resilience in order that we develop a comfort zone, from which we can respond to, and deal with, stressful events as they arise. The first step that we need to take along this path involves exploring and understanding the differences between positive and negative stress.

Sleeping with the Enemy: Taming Negative Stress

The following scenario – or a variation on it – may be all too familiar to many of us. We have been out too late, drunk too much on an empty stomach after a demanding day at work, and arrived home feeling the worse for wear. As a result, the next morning we oversleep and have to rush off to work feeling grouchy, hardly awake and ill-prepared to meet the demands of the day. We grab a couple of painkillers as a quick fix for a growing, nagging headache, without taking the time to have the drink of water that we desperately need to deal with the dehydration that is making the headache worse.

Because we are leaving later than usual, we may find that we get snarled up in a traffic jam that normally, leaving at an earlier time, we would avoid. As we stagger into work we are likely to be feeling even more out of sorts and short-fused than we were, and, what is worse, looking rough. By mid-morning we feel like we are wading through treacle, so we grab a quick, strong coffee before we go into an important meeting and sneak a chocolate fix with it — why shouldn't we? This provides us with a temporary lift, but when the effect wears off (much

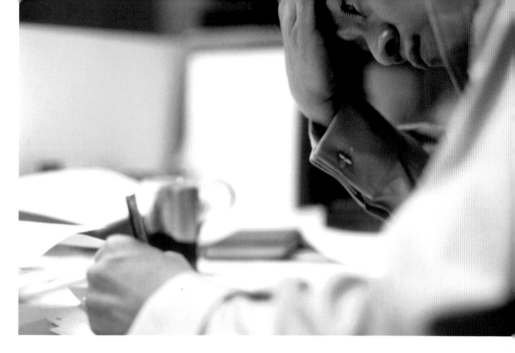

more quickly than we would have expected), the headache is probably worse and any degree of concentration is a huge problem. So when we are asked for our contribution to the meeting, we end up feeling completely out of our depth.

By lunchtime all we really want to do is go home and sleep. Instead we end up eating more comfort food because we feel so miserable. Then, having consumed a packet of crisps, a bacon sandwich and another bar of chocolate, we feel sick and even more frustrated with ourselves. We drag ourselves back to work where, because this has turned into the 'day from hell', we start snapping at anyone who has the temerity to come near us. Well aware of what is going on, we long to go home and start again.

By the time we actually open our front door we remember with a groan the mess that is about to greet us: all the boring jobs that we have been putting on hold. All we want is to be magically transported to a fragrant, mess-free, ordered zone with a full refrigerator and a favourite CD playing softly in the background.

Extreme and predictable though this scenario may seem, most of us, if we are honest, will not be strangers to some of its painful elements. The point of describing this 'day from hell' is to show how, by

reacting in a different way, many of the stressful factors could have been avoided altogether, or their effects at least reduced considerably. This, then, becomes a working example of how stress can be buffered and managed if we are prepared to meet it, and if we know what lifestyle choices can turn stress from a burden into a blessing. Most important of all, we will come to appreciate the vital fact that stress itself can be neutral: it is the way in which we react to it that ultimately determines whether it becomes a negative or a positive influence.

Going with the Flow: Making Friends with Positive Stress

We can take the first step towards understanding how we can meet stress on an equal and effective footing if we stop and reprise the 'day from hell' from a subtly altered perspective.

We know that tomorrow morning we have an important meeting when we will need to be on particularly sharp form, so we make sure that we do

13

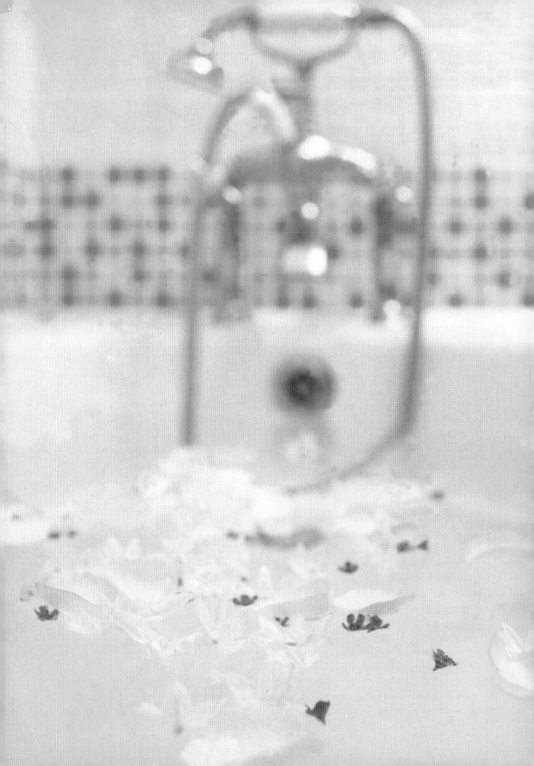

not take up a casual invitation at short notice to go out for a few drinks after work. Instead we arrange to meet at the weekend, when we know we can let our hair down without worrying about any knock-on effects at work the next day.

By getting home early we have time to run (and soak in) a warm bath scented with invigorating aromatherapy oils, from which we emerge feeling perked up and ready for the evening ahead. This gives us the chance to catch up on some work after dinner in preparation for the important meeting the following day – although, in order that we give ourselves the opportunity to switch off completely and get a sound night's sleep, we must avoid the temptation to continue to work into the early hours.

Because we are starting the day feeling refreshed and relaxed, if we do find ourselves caught in an unexpected traffic jam the next morning, it does not cause us to become 'wired' and short-fused. Instead, because we feel positive and in command, we choose to use the extra time spent in the snarl-up to listen to a CD, a favourite that always makes us feel happy. Once we get to work, a cup of green tea will get us off to a clear-headed and energized start to the day.

By the time of the mid-morning meeting we feel composed and articulate about what we want to contribute. It goes even better than expected, so that, by lunchtime, we feel great. As a result, when it comes to food, we make a healthy choice: salad with a wholemeal roll, lots of fresh fruit to follow, and a bottle of mineral water with a twist of lemon. The delicious cup of fresh coffee that we order to round it off is an indulgence we can easily afford, because the basic framework of our day thus far has been full of positive, healthy options.

For the rest of the day, because we feel relaxed and confident, others see us as approachable and this benefits the overall atmosphere. By the time we get home we feel ready for a relaxing bath, a glass of wine – only one, of course! – and a couple of hours in front of a favourite video.

left SOAKING FOR A WHILE IN A WARM BATH IS A LOVELY WAY OF INDUCING A RELAXED STATE.

How to Achieve and Maintain Balance

As with so many things in life, what we are essentially aiming for in stress management is establishing a point of optimum balance. Once we have identified this ideal state, we should discover that we have enough positive stress in our daily lives to keep us motivated and focused, but also enough built-in relaxation space within which to unwind and recharge our emotional, mental and physical batteries.

If we take the imaginary scenarios in the section above as working examples, we can see that what we are striving for is a healthy balance between control and spontaneity. In other words, if we take the second, positive scenario and apply its principles in a more rigid and extreme way, we are likely to end up being just as stressed as we were in the first, negative scenario, because we will find that our life becomes excessively ordered and obsessive. Moreover, most of our colleagues and friends are likely, quite quickly, to become thoroughly sick and tired of having to deal with a saint in their midst, so it will be a regime that is isolating as well.

The negative scenario, on the other hand, has tipped the balance in too extreme a way in the other direction: healthy spontaneity has moved into the zone where it promotes a sequence of negative events that, in a domino effect, raise stress levels. As we can see, this has no benefits for friends, colleagues or family either, because, as a result of feeling under constant, excessive pressure, we are likely to suffer from rollercoasting mood swings.

Thus the essential difference between negative and positive stress can be summed up as follows. Negative stress leaves us feeling fraught, unable to come close to meeting the demands with which we are presented, powerless, indecisive, irritable and fearful (this last to a degree that can often seem disproportionate to its trigger). Positive stress, on the other hand, promotes the opposite mental and emotional reaction, so that, among other things, we feel decisive, energized, comfortably in command of the situation we are asked to meet, and exhilarated.

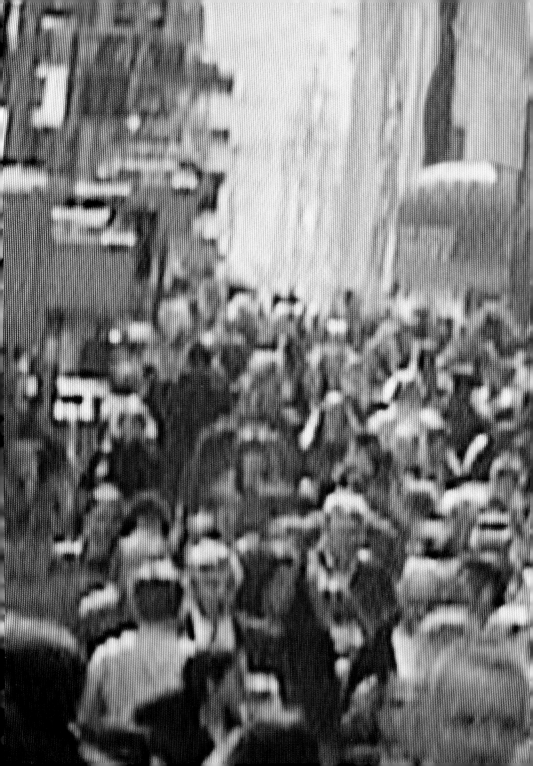

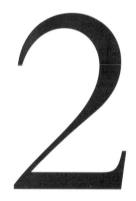

2 Under Pressure: Negative Effects of Stress on the Mind, Emotions and Body

This popular reaction is underpinned and bolstered by the messages we pick up from newspapers, magazines, television and the Internet. Collaboratively, these media present a persuasive case, suggesting that we are effectively, today, experiencing an epidemic of stress-related illnesses. These health problems are alarmingly wide-ranging in nature, and have been shown to have an extremely negative effect on our mental, emotional and physical wellbeing and equilibrium. Stress-related physical problems can, as a result, have a detrimental effect on our personal and professional relationships, making us feel even more stressed and therefore at the mercy of negative events.

Some of us are so tuned in to our bodies that we can register quite rapidly the characteristic sensations and changes in our bodies that are known to be

left THE HECTIC PACE OF MODERN CITY LIFE CAN PLAY A MAJOR ROLE IN GENERATING WHATEVER FEELINGS WE MAY HAVE OF BEING UNDER PRESSURE.

direct responses to exposure to an excessive negative stress load: anything from an awareness of a dry mouth, sweaty palms, or rapid and shallow breathing, to a feeling of slight queasiness or light-headedness. There are indeed specific symptoms that develop when we are under stress, some of which can be still subtler signs and sensations than those just listed. If we are to learn how to manage stress as effectively and positively as possible, it is essential to be able to identify these symptoms and to understand the mechanism that triggers them.

As with so many other situations in life, we can find effective solutions only when we understand fully the nature of the problem. This is especially true of any discussion of stress management. We need to understand why our bodies react in a specific way to pressure and stress. Once we do this, we can better support our minds, emotions and bodies in dealing with whatever problems we face in as balanced, energized and positive a way as possible.

Always bear in mind that a feeling of being powerless to change our situation will lead us to feel even more stressed and trapped in a negative spiral of symptoms. On the other hand, simply by applying stress-reduction techniques we are taking a degree of control into our own hands – and this act alone can do a huge amount to relieve the pressure of unresolved stress.

The Stress Response and How to Live with it

Here we owe a great deal to Hans Seyle. Often referred to as the 'father of stress', in the 1930s Seyle was the first scientist to examine the concept of stress in relation to human behaviour. The stress reaction explored by Seyle has been referred to as the general adaptation syndrome (GAS, for short). In a state of good health the basic function of GAS is to maintain a condition of optimum balance (often called homeostasis), so that the whole system is not drastically thrown off balance at any given time.

Any stressor that comes into contact with our bodies has the potential seriously to threaten homeostasis. And stressors can appear in a bewildering array of situations, from shock, and being involved in or witnessing an accident, to receiving exciting news; from bereavement to pregnancy; from redundancy, or a deadline at work that we will have to push ourselves to meet, to contracting a serious illness, or falling foul of postnatal depression, or suffering from extreme anxiety.

Whatever the nature of the stressor, as soon as our bodies become aware of its presence, we move into an initial stage of arousal. This is followed rapidly by a stage of activity during which a whole range of physiological mechanisms designed to meet the perceived stressor are mobilized. We will experience,

below **BY LEARNING HOW TO SWITCH ON THE RELAXATION RESPONSE WE WILL BE ABLE TO RELAX AT WILL WHEREVER WE ARE, IN ANY CIRCUMSTANCES.**

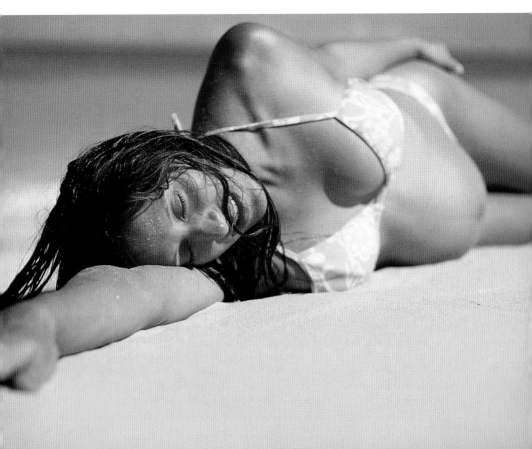

to begin with, a phase of increased mental and physical energy, coupled with symptoms of physical tension. If, however, this phase continues for an excessive period, or is not succeeded by a phase of effective mental and physical relaxation, we will move into the final stage: exhaustion, where chronic fatigue can become a severe problem.

Although these principles can be generally applied, it is also very important to bear in mind that each of us will respond to what we perceive as stressful in our own unique way. Some people appear to adapt much more easily to pressure and change than others; they may positively welcome some stresses that others regard as a negative experience. Looking at people's reactions to an event such as moving house provides us with a simple, practical example of how some of us have more adaptive resources and resilience than others.

Some of us find it necessary to move house frequently for the stimulation, the challenge and the excitement it engenders. For those who find that they must have the basic security and order of their home in a settled and stable state in order to function at their best in social and professional settings, however, this would be a hellish scenario.

Providing that neither example is taken to an extreme, we could quite accurately conclude from this that the house-mover has more adaptive energy than the homebird, and is likely to be able to roll with the punches of everyday stress with more resilience and ease. Nevertheless, it must also be borne in mind that even those who readily embrace the challenge and exhilaration of change can unwittingly reach the point of exhaustion if they are not on the lookout for early warning signs of burnout.

The 'Fight-or-Flight' Response

Whenever we are faced with a stressful situation, our bodies respond by initiating a rapid-response technique, aptly known as the 'fight-or-flight' reaction – punch the tiger in the jaws, or run for it! The basic function of this rapidly triggered response is to allow us to take prompt and decisive physical action in the face of a threatening situation. Any changes that occur are designed to support us as we engage in whatever response is appropriate to meeting the crisis – from actively engaging in physical combat, to sprinting to safety away from the presence of the threat, as the name suggests.

In order to allow us to take either course of action, our bodies undergo a series of involuntary changes. Blood-sugar levels are raised to provide us with extra energy; there is increased secretion of adrenaline and cortisol (both known to be potent stress hormones), which raises our blood pressure and makes our heart beat faster; breathing accelerates and becomes shallower; digestive activity is virtually shut down, leading to a strong impulse to empty the bowels or regurgitate the contents of the stomach; and muscles receive an augmented blood supply in order to make a speedy sprint away from danger more possible.

Allowing us to take almost immediate physical action when we are confronted by a dangerous or threatening situation, this is a very effective protective mechanism. If we have to trigger the fight-or-flight reaction regularly, however, even if each occasion warrants only a low-grade response, serious health problems will inevitably arise.

If our bodies are activating this inbuilt stress-related mechanism every time we receive an unexpectedly large bill, have a fight with our partner, feel that our colleagues are being unnecessarily critical, or have to give one of a series of regular presentations at work, it is more or less inevitable that we will suffer unpleasant consequences. These can include anything from indigestion, irritable bowel syndrome, high blood pressure, insomnia, anxiety, unstable blood-sugar levels and muscle pain to tension headaches or migraines.

As some of these events are unavoidable features of everyday life, there is little point in wishing that they would disappear. The secret of effective stress management lies in discovering the specific techniques that suit us as individuals, so that we find ways of recovering rapidly from the fight-or-flight response, and effectively switch off from its negative consequences. In order to do this, we need to have a working knowledge of how the autonomic nervous system functions.

The Autonomic Nervous System

The autonomic nervous system is implicated in a staggeringly wide range of basic bodily functions that are classed as involuntary. In other words, we do not consciously have to do anything in order either to initiate or to alter any of these activities. They include changes of blood pressure; stimulating the flow of digestive juices in order to promote smooth digestive function; regulating the heartbeat; promoting perspiration to cool us down when we are overheated; and physical changes that come about as a result of sexual arousal. Obviously, then, the autonomic nervous system can be regarded as a key player in the maintenance of effective homeostasis.

The autonomic nervous system comprises two branches with directly opposing functions: the sympathetic and the parasympathetic. Together they provide us with an elegant example of how a perfect whole, working at peak efficiency, may be made up of two opposing forces working in a balanced way.

The sympathetic wing of the autonomic system is tuned in to the fight-or-flight response, because it is made up of a group of nerve fibres that are involved with adrenaline secretion. As a result, the sympathetic branch triggers nervous energy, preparing us to meet physical, emotional and mental challenges (including tigers) by stimulating a rapid heartbeat, accelerating our breathing, promoting perspiration, raising the blood pressure, shutting down the secretion of gastric juices, and sending extra blood to the muscles so that they are ready for action.

The function of the parasympathetic wing, on the other hand, is to help us to relax or chill out after a major challenge. It is the part of the autonomic nervous system that promotes recovery from the stress response. Not surprisingly, then, the parasympathetic branch is responsible for slowing down the resting heartbeat, regulating smooth respiration, kickstarting effective digestion, and promoting muscle relaxation. A protracted period of stress, when we feel constantly tense, edgy and strung up, will force us to enter a zone where the sympathetic nervous system is dominant. In contrast, those of us who feel laidback most of the time, and who can recover quickly from periods of short-term stress, are reaping the benefits of an efficiently functioning parasympathetic nervous system.

In effective stress management we are striving to adopt a lifestyle that encourages optimum balance between the two opposing branches of the autonomic nervous system. If and when we achieve this, we will no longer need to rely on the bustle and buzz of a high-pressure lifestyle to make us feel alive and energized.

As we have already seen, an imbalance towards the sympathetic wing may well fill us with a feeling of adrenaline-fuelled nervous energy in the short term, but we will pay a very high price in the health stakes if we rely on this energy for too long. In addition, too much stress for too long leaves us hooked on the adrenaline surge, and before long we will find ourselves mentally, emotionally and physically exhausted.

Being excessively laidback and relaxed also has its pitfalls, however: life may seem to lose its stimulating edge, for instance. If we have too few challenges to meet, we run the risk of becoming unmotivated, sluggish and bored. This in itself can turn into a different sort of stress that we will also need to avoid if we are to get the most out of life.

Believe it or not, we all benefit from being pushed to meet deadlines, whether these take the form of getting physically fit in preparation for pregnancy, revising for an important exam, getting psyched up for an interview, or writing a book that has to be delivered by a specific date in order for a tight publishing schedule to run smoothly. It has been said that nothing focuses the mind like a non-negotiable deadline, and, in my own experience, this is absolutely true. From a different perspective, without a healthy degree of stress, life would undoubtedly lose its spice.

Achieving the Balance

In the past it was thought that we were unable to influence involuntary functions such as fluctuations in blood pressure, heartbeat and body temperature (precisely because they are not under the conscious control of the body). In fact, research with yoga practitioners and using deep-meditation techniques has shown that during profound states of relaxation subjects can, by conscious control, dramatically lower their blood pressure, heartbeat, respiration rates and body temperature.

Some of these studies are discussed by Dr Herbert Benson in his books: *The Relaxation Response* and *Beyond The Relaxation Response*. The revelation that through conscious control we can have an impact on a body system that was previously thought to be unreachable (the parasympathetic branch of the nervous system) has opened up a variety of extremely positive possibilities for those of us who need to find effective stress-management techniques. Chapter Three will teach us more about achieving conscious relaxation.

Other important lifestyle factors that have been shown to have a measurable effect on stress and its reduction include nutrition and exercise. Ironically, in a high-stress lifestyle these are often the first elements to suffer, because many of us feel that we really do not have the time or energy to devote ourselves to eating well or getting fit. Chapters Three and Four will explain what a disastrous approach this is, illustrating

below AS WELL AS PROMOTING A DEEP SENSE OF RELAXATION, MEDITATION ALSO IMPROVES CONCENTRATION.

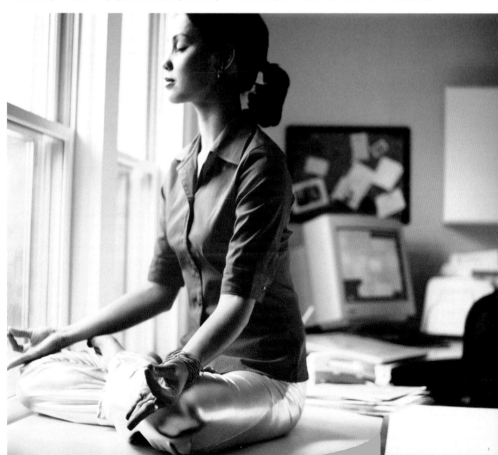

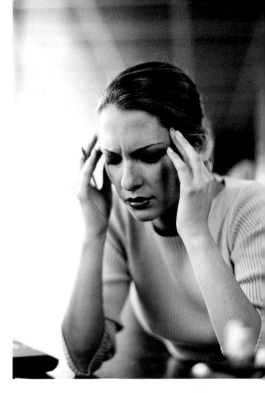

how, by becoming a couch potato and relying on quick-fix foods, we are virtually asking stress-related symptoms to become an established part of our lives.

Despite our best intentions, life will go off the rails for all of us from time to time. Chapter Seven is designed to help if a short-term, stress-related problem does arise within the context of a generally sound lifestyle. A wide range of alternative and complementary therapies that will get us back on track as quickly as possible are suggested.

By following the advice in the following chapters we will be putting into operation a total de-stress plan. As a consequence, we will maximize our energy and vitality to meet positive stress head on, while exploring ways of relaxing our whole system on all levels – mental, emotional and physical.

Before we embark on this exciting journey towards de-stressing ourselves, we need to identify our particular problem areas as regards stress. In order to do this, we need to determine the most common symptoms and triggers of stress.

Identifying Stress

Excessive negative stress that is not dealt with effectively will give rise to certain signs and symptoms – early warning signals that all is not well.

GENERAL SYMPTOMS

Any of the following may be regarded as general symptoms:

- Overall muscular tension with particular discomfort and stiffness in the jaw, neck and shoulders
- Lack of zest for life
- Insomnia or poor-quality, fitful sleep
- Wandering or poorly focused concentration
- Fatigue
- Lowered libido
- Recurrent infections – anything from frequent colds to skin outbreaks
- Poor appetite

MENTAL AND EMOTIONAL SYMPTOMS

These, commonly triggered by an excess of negative stress, can include any of the following:

- Anxiety
- Panic attacks
- Depression
- Lack of confidence
- Indecision
- Rapid or unpredictable mood swings
- Inability to switch off after work

PHYSICAL SYMPTOMS

These tend to appear as a result of stress – singly or together, or in quick succession – and can include:

- Indigestion
- Heartburn
- Diarrhoea
- Constipation
- Tension headaches
- Hyperventilation (rapid, shallow breathing)
- Palpitations (consciousness of a fluttering, irregular or unnaturally fast heartbeat)

- Dizziness and light-headedness
- Tingling sensations or pins and needles

BEHAVIOURAL SYMPTOMS

Unfortunately, we can also unwittingly make stress-related problems worse for ourselves by adopting short-term strategies for coping that, in themselves, have further negative effects on our health. These can be called behavioural symptoms. Such strategies can include any combination of the following:

- Increased consumption of alcohol
- Smoking
- Overuse of prescription drugs, such as painkillers
- Use of recreational drugs
- Overreliance on caffeinated drinks to keep energy levels high
- Increased consumption of sugar and chocolate
- Comfort eating

LONG-TERM PHYSICAL EFFECTS

If exposure to unacceptably high stress levels goes on for an extended period of time without strategies being in place for managing this pressure effectively, the scene is set for the emergence of more long-term health problems. These can include any combination of the following:

- Migraines and recurrent headaches
- Irritable bowel syndrome
- Clinical depression
- Chronic anxiety
- Phobias
- Permanent pain, or a lack of mobility and stiffness in the neck and shoulders
- Stomach ulcers
- Eczema
- Psoriasis
- Reduced function of the immune system, giving rise to the potential for anything from persistent colds to established cystitis; and the likely aggravation of more chronic inflammatory conditions, such as rheumatoid arthritis

right ANY SHORT-TERM PLEASURE DERIVED FROM COMFORT EATING IS QUITE LIKELY, OVER A LONGER PERIOD, TO BE REPLACED BY DIGESTIVE PROBLEMS AND FATIGUE.

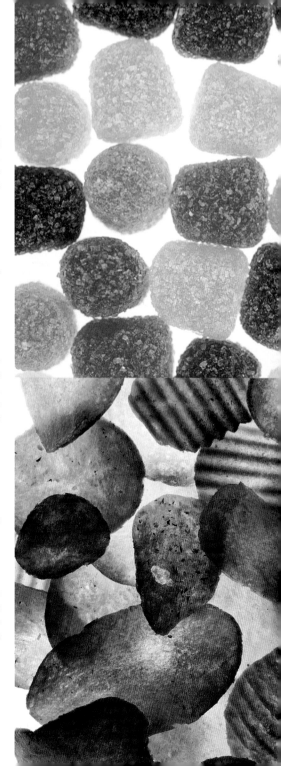

Sources of Excessive Stress

Any situation can become a source of negative stress if we perceive it to be threatening or out of our control – as we have already seen. There are also a number of common triggers of unwelcome stress, however, which are especially powerful if they occur simultaneously or in very quick succession. To divide these into two basic groups – interpersonal and professional stressors – is convenient and helpful.

INTERPERSONAL STRESSORS
- Lack of communication
- Unexpressed anger
- Lack of physical contact
- Financial pressures
- Low self-esteem
- Guilt
- Anxiety
- Depression
- Isolation and loneliness
- Boredom
- Absence of sense of humour

PROFESSIONAL STRESSORS
- Poor time-management skills
- Inability to delegate
- Absence of good organization in the working environment
- Lack of motivation
- Sick building syndrome
- Noise
- Unrealistic goals and targets
- Drab surroundings

It is really crucial to realize that however daunting these two lists might appear, there is positive action that can be taken to deal with each of the stressors listed. And when we appreciate that action is the primary key to stress-busting, we will be free to break out from the cage where we feel hopeless and helpless.

First of all we must prioritize, identifying the issues that are causing us the most pressure and stress.

Putting De-stress Principles into Practice

Before we look at strategies for dealing with particular groups of stress-related problems, this seems an appropriate moment to discuss in greater detail the structure and format of the de-stress plan. It has five major sections:
- Calm
- Nourish
- Replenish
- Pamper
- Rebalance

Calm is a section that speaks for itself. It is devoted to exploring the basic mental and emotional techniques that we can – and should – employ to take control and defuse stress from within.

Nourish deals with the known links between stress and diet, and shows us how to break free from those eating/drinking habits that can actively contribute to extra strain in our lives.

Replenish explores exercise techniques that are known to calm both the mind and emotions, while stimulating a balanced, sustained release of energy.

Pamper – in many ways my favourite section, because it deals with an area that is often neglected in more spartan approaches to health promotion – is devoted to describing techniques that will provide us with a stress-free comfort zone to use at home.

Rebalance looks at the use of complementary and alternative medicine in the treatment of stress.

Taking the First Step: Identifying Our Priorities

If most of our problems appear among the mental and emotional symptoms and are echoed in the list of interpersonal stressors, we will benefit greatly from the advice given in the Calm and Rebalance sections.

Those of us who are primarily concerned with physical and behavioural problems need to look in detail at the Nourish and Rebalance sections.

Others, who feel their concerns are more diffuse and can be categorized as general symptoms, may find that following the advice in the Replenish and Pamper sections makes a radical difference.

Do bear in mind that these are only suggestions, not engraved in stone, and that each section may be used as creatively as you feel is appropriate. Always remember that whatever advice you take on board must feel right for your individual needs, tastes and temperament. Above all, remember that having fun can only ever be beneficial. Be creative with some of these suggestions.

Dealing Effectively with Long-Term Stress-Related Problems

The stress-related problems that appear under the heading of long-term physical effects demand separate consideration, for while the self-help advice given in the de-stress plan can ameliorate many of the conditions listed, there are also some problems that should be treated by a trained complementary or alternative therapist. Chronic medical conditions (as those listed here generally are) fall into this category.

Home-prescribers can quickly find themselves out of their depth with chronic conditions, which, by their very nature, tend to be well established and often complex in nature. The situation will be further complicated if conventional medication is being taken, because it is often difficult for a newcomer to self-prescribing to discern whether symptoms are connected to the original complaint or are side effects of the medication.

Anyone suffering from recurrent migraines, clinical depression, psoriasis, established anxiety, eczema, stomach ulcers or irritable bowel syndrome may like to seek alternative medical advice. It is very important to stress, though, that if conventional drugs are being used to treat any of these conditions, they should never be discontinued unless under medical supervision or with medical advice.

Appropriate therapies would include homeopathy, Western medical herbalism and traditional Chinese medicine. Aromatherapy, hypnotherapy, reflexology and massage would provide complementary help.

For anyone struggling with a chronic, stress-related problem, it can be especially helpful to consult an alternative medical practitioner because of the way that alternative approaches to healing work from the premise that the body possesses its own inbuilt, self-balancing and self-regulating mechanism. Alternative medical treatment, such as homeopathy, is aimed at stimulating the whole system to regain its optimum point of equilibrium. From what we have learnt about stress-related problems being the result of an upset in this balance, it is clear that a system of healing that has maintaining homeostasis as its primary objective is likely to be particularly suitable.

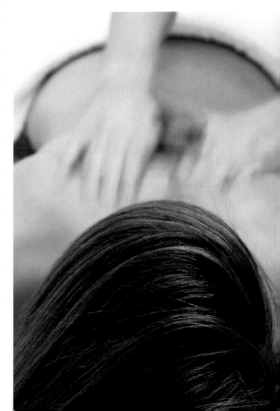

right A REGULAR NECK AND SHOULDER MASSAGE CAN BE VERY HELPFUL IN EASING HEADACHES THAT ARE TRIGGERED BY TENSION AROUND THE BASE OF THE NECK.

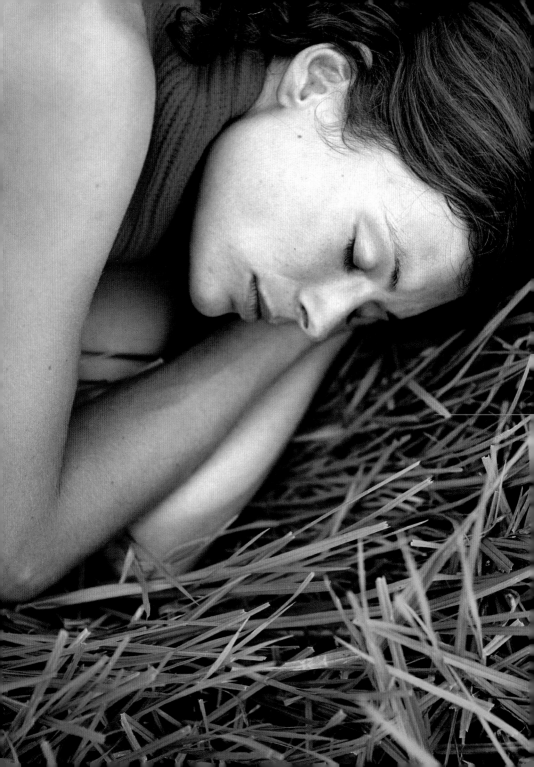

3 Calm: Relaxing the Body and Soothing the Soul

If we stop to consider just how much bustle and noise surrounds us daily, it is astonishing that we manage to concentrate on anything. Insistently ringing telephones, blaring radios, raised voices, yelling children, alarms going off unexpectedly and flight paths overhead all contribute to the busy general hum of life.

If, while we are already struggling to meet a tight deadline at work, we heap on to this contextual stress the additional layer of pressure contributed by the ubiquitous use of fax, email and cell phones, is there any wonder that there are times when we want to shut the door on everything, and wander away to our private oasis of calm and serenity?

This chapter is about exactly that. If we regularly apply the practical advice that follows, we will be able to access a serene retreat – without having to remove ourselves from the source of our stress. All we need to do, in order to be able to induce a state of mental and emotional calm whenever we sense the unmistakable early warning signs of developing tension and strain, is master some basic skills. And knowing that the relaxation response can be switched

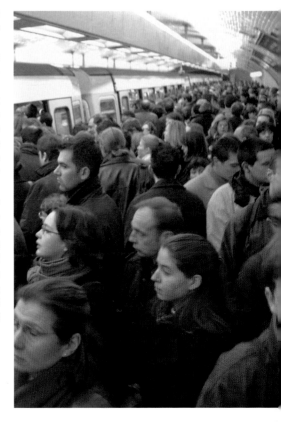

left FOR MANY OF US, 'CHILLING OUT' IS A LEARNT RATHER THAN AN INSTINCTIVE SKILL. right GET UP 15 MINUTES EARLIER THAN NECESSARY TO GIVE YOURSELF ENOUGH TIME FOR A QUIET AND UNHURRIED START TO THE DAY, WHICH WILL STRENGTHEN YOU TO COPE WITH THE PRESSURES OF TRAVEL.

on at will is likely to provide a significant sense of security and empowerment. This is particularly important if we live or work in an environment that is full of bustle, because there is nothing quite so calming and stress-reducing as feeling that we can take the situation into our own hands and control it.

Some of the techniques are designed to be practised regularly at home, becoming an established part of our lives. Others are suggested as quasi 'quick fixes'; they can be used wherever we are to defuse an evolving stressful situation without delay.

In the de-stress plan, we are ideally aiming to include regular sessions of some form of relaxation technique, to create a healthy baseline of calm. By positively influencing the long term in this way, we are likely to discover that we do not have to rely so much on the quick fixes as damage-limitation strategies.

Switching Off Stress

Dr Herbert Benson, in his book *The Relaxation Response*, provides us with a powerful antidote to the fight-or-flight response described in the previous chapter. As we have seen, the physical changes that are triggered by the fight-or-flight response are intimately interlinked with increased activity of the sympathetic nervous system.

Too much stimulation in this direction will inevitably cause symptoms of jitteriness, anxiety, aggression, rapid heartbeat, insomnia and light-headedness (as a result of rapid, shallow breathing). These, of course, are just the tip of a tension-filled

below **BEDROOMS SHOULD BE QUIET, WELL VENTILATED AND DARK ENOUGH TO HELP INDUCE A REFRESHING NIGHT'S SLEEP.**

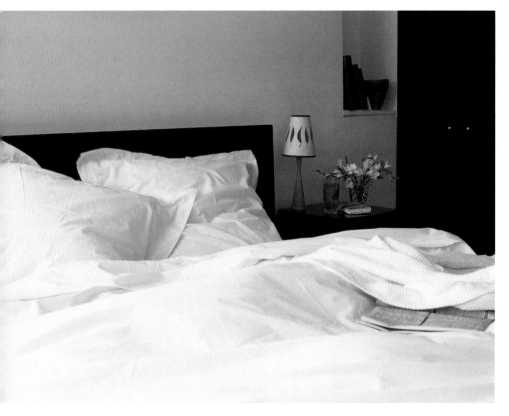

iceberg; a number of subtler, less obviously detectable changes will be happening at the same time, which will leave us vulnerable to any number of the chronic, stress-related problems outlined in the previous chapter.

However, we do have at our disposal the relaxation response, which is an effective method of initiating an antidote to increased activity of the sympathetic nervous system. Whether it is triggered through meditation, progressive muscular relaxation, creative visualization, biofeedback, autogenic training, or relaxation techniques, the relaxation response appears to prompt physical responses characteristic of stimulated parasympathetic nervous system activity.

There are several signs that indicate that the parasympathetic nervous system is being brought into play: decreased oxygen consumption, a lowered heart rate, slower respiration and a marked decrease in blood-lactate levels. The latter is significant because high blood-lactate levels are associated with anxiety-related symptoms. When we activate the relaxation response, in other words, we move into a profoundly restful state of being.

It is important to understand, however, that while parallels can be drawn between the physiological changes that occur in induced relaxation and in the sleeping state (such as a decreased consumption of oxygen), the experience of deep relaxation is not the same as sleep. Thus we cannot just assume that because we are getting regular, sound, good-quality sleep, we are automatically reaping the same benefits as we would from the relaxation response.

One of the important differences between the two activities relates to the presence of alpha (slow) brain waves. Not, as a rule, found during sleep, alpha waves do characterize deep relaxation, together with some other brain-wave activity. Conversely, the brain-wave signals associated with rapid-eye movement (REM) sleep and dreaming are absent in meditation.

Although deep relaxation and sleep are different, the importance of regular, refreshing sleep should never be ignored in any discussion of stress-management techniques. Healthy patterns of sleep help guard against low energy levels, mood swings and recurrent infections.

Relaxation for the Long Term: Basic Practicalities

Before exploring some of the basic techniques available to us for effective de-stressing, it is equally important to look at some of the practical issues we will need to consider if we are trying to practise relaxation at home. After all, it is unlikely that we will enjoy the pleasure of relaxation or reap its benefits if we are in any way uncomfortable.

WARMTH
It may come as a surprise to a novice to discover that our body temperature can drop significantly during a state of deep relaxation. To avoid feeling at all uncomfortably chilled, always make sure at the beginning of a session that your surroundings are warm enough.

CLARITY
Equally, though, avoid the temptation to make the environment too hot and stuffy, as this can induce sleepiness rather than a state of relaxation. If this happens, there is a risk that, rather than emerging from relaxation clear-headed and serene, you will wake feeling groggy and disoriented.

COMFORT
It does pay to give some attention to what we wear during a relaxation exercise, though it is not necessary to invest in special fitness clothes. The most important thing is to find something in which we feel totally at ease: anything from a combination of tracksuit bottoms and a warm T-shirt or sweatshirt to a favourite cosy, long, loose dress. The main points to consider are a lack of restriction – around the neck, wrists and waist – and soft fabric that feels soothing and pleasurable on the skin.

PROPS
If relaxing in an upright, sitting position, always choose a straight-backed chair to give the spine maximum support. Hunching or slouching has the undesirable effect of making the breathing shallower. Sitting comfortably upright, on the other hand,

automatically encourages the contents of the chest cavity to expand more effectively. Make sure that the feet are also positioned as comfortably as possible, checking that the soles of your feet rest easily and firmly on the surface of the floor. Your hands can lie either in your lap or on the arms of the chair.

If you choose to be lying down to relax, use a surface that is flat and comfortably firm; an exercise mat or a folded blanket on the floor work equally well in this respect.

PEACE

Always make sure that background noise will be kept to a minimum before starting a practice session. Switch the telephone to answering-machine mode, and as far as is feasible switch off any other appliance that is likely to make an unexpected noise. And remember to tell the rest of the family what you are doing in advance, so that you minimize the chances of being disturbed.

REGULARITY

As with any form of discipline, the hardest part is likely to be establishing a habit of regular practice. However, the benefits of relaxation appear to depend heavily on regular practice – whatever technique is followed. So aim to build some conscious relaxation time into each day, although a day or two without a session does not warrant getting stressed about. After all, this would just defeat the object of what you are attempting to do in the first place. Instead, just resume your relaxation practice as though there had been no interruption, and enjoy afresh the benefits it brings.

TEMPERAMENT AND LIFESTYLE

If regular practice of conscious relaxation is going to become an integral part of your daily routine, it is essential to choose a method that you feel is appropriate to you as an individual. If you have an instinctive dislike of gadgets and electronic devices, for example, you are not likely to find biofeedback appealing. You would do better to choose a technique that requires no specialized equipment and can be applied with ease in any situation where you may feel stressed and under undue pressure.

Autogenic Training

This is a system of medical therapy developed by a German neurologist called Dr Schultz. Once learnt, the technique should be practised every day in order to induce a state of calm and relaxation. Autogenic training involves focusing the mind on six mental exercises that relate to initiating and identifying specific sensations in parts of the body.

In order to tackle the training it is helpful to lie down in quiet surroundings with your eyes shut. Once you have mastered the technique, you can use it anywhere, at any time, to withdraw into a voluntary state of tranquillity.

Each exercise focuses the mind on actively experiencing in the limbs a variety of sensations (heaviness, coolness or warmth), while remaining aware of heart rate and breathing rhythms.

It is advisable to be trained by a skilled teacher in autogenic training rather than trying to master the technique alone. Occasionally psychological reactions, such as an increase in anxiety, can occur in response to autogenic training, and if this should happen it is extremely helpful to have the support of a skilled and experienced practitioner on standby to evaluate what is happening and to act swiftly and intelligently upon that analysis.

Once the basic exercises have been learnt, autogenic training can be used to induce a deeply relaxed state within a relatively short timescale. However, do remember that if you want to experience the keen sense of observation that develops as you gradually learn to become aware of different physical sensations in a state of deep relaxation, regular practice is essential. Repetition is vital, both as regards the exercises themselves and the key phrases that form the structure of the training. Your perseverance will be rewarded by the benefits that flow from this valuable therapy.

right TRY TO BUILD TIME FOR RELAXATION INTO EACH DAY, TO RE-CREATE THE SENSE OF RELEASE WE ENJOY ON HOLIDAYS.

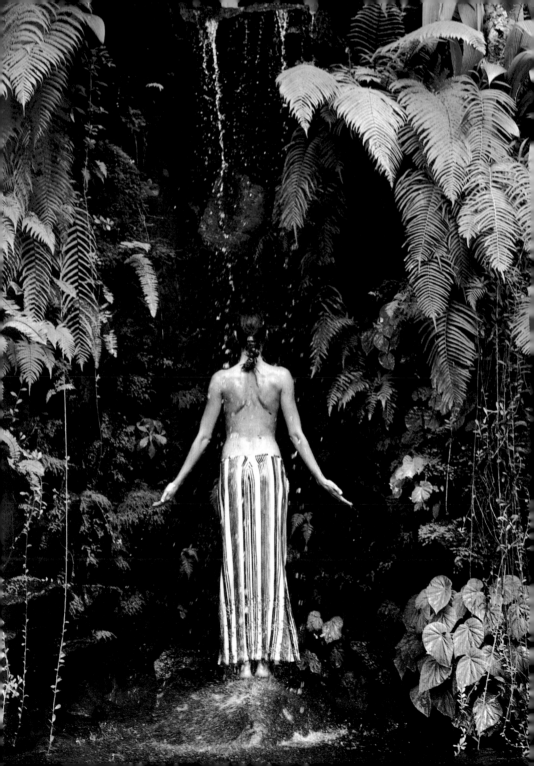

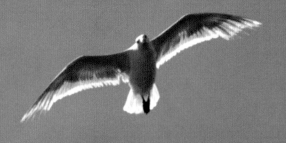

Progressive Muscular Relaxation

This is a technique that involves the cumulative, conscious relaxation of muscle groups. The system was devised by a physiologist called Dr Jacobson, who considered that states of anxiety and mental and emotional tension could be triggered or made more intense by muscular contraction or tightness. He also came to the conclusion that the reverse was equally true. In other words, practising regular, voluntary muscular relaxation could actively contribute to the establishment of a sense of mental and emotional calm and tranquillity.

The technique involves consciously tightening up a group of muscles (clenching our hands into fists, for example), holding the contraction for a second or two, and then consciously relaxing them and very deliberately letting the muscles go as fully as possible. The effect can be enhanced if you envisage that you are letting go of all the worries you are carrying as you release the muscle tension in each part of the body in turn.

It is also helpful to become conscious of the pattern and rhythm of your breathing as you practise progressive muscular relaxation (PMR). Inhaling fully through the nose as you tighten the muscle groups, you should then exhale deeply through the mouth – with a sigh – as the muscles are relaxed and softened.

PMR needs to be practised regularly, lying down in a quiet room. As you become proficient in the technique, you are likely to become aware of when you are holding even the smallest amount of muscular contraction in the face and eyes, as well as in the larger muscle groups of the arms and legs. By identifying these contractions and being able to let go of them at will, you can achieve a profound state of relaxation.

left BY CONSCIOUSLY RELAXING OUR MUSCLES WE CAN INDUCE A PROFOUND SENSE OF MENTAL AND EMOTIONAL TRANQUILLITY, AND FEEL LIKE A BIRD SOARING IN THE SKY.

Biofeedback

The use of biofeedback dates back to the 1960s. It was then that US scientists became aware of the positive potential of biofeedback devices in their treatment of patients needing to control stress-related problems, such as high blood pressure.

The patient is linked up by electrodes and probes to a biofeedback machine. Once a session is under way, information is fed back to the patient about changes in his or her body (variations in heart rate and muscle tension) through beeps, flashes or moving needles on a dial on the biofeedback device.

The basic changes that are monitored by biofeedback include variations in the skin's heat levels, the amount of perspiration produced, the degree of muscle tension present, brain-wave activity and variations in the heart rate. A relaxed state is associated with an absence of excess perspiration, high levels of alpha waves and a regular, slow heart rate, so the monitored results provide the patients with objective information about how relaxed or not they may be.

Over a period of time, patients become aware of how conscious control – though breathing techniques and muscle relaxation – can have a beneficial effect when they are inducing a state of relaxation. As a result, they are empowered to reduce troublesome stress symptoms, such as anxiety and muscle tension. There are some problems that seem to respond especially well to biofeedback training; these include tension headaches, migraines, high blood pressure, irritable bowel syndrome and insomnia.

Meditation

Exponents of meditation are extremely enthusiastic about the way in which, practised regularly, it can reduce a formidably wide range of stress-related problems that we battle with often. As well as helping those who suffer from anxiety, insomnia, high blood pressure and recurrent problems as a result of muscle tension, regular practice of meditation appears significantly to improve levels of concentration and to focus the mind, making us generally more creative, single-minded and productive. This sense of purpose means that energy is not squandered in endless worrying and anxiety, so it could also be argued that meditation confers the additional bonus of being able to regulate energy levels.

Meditation has been described as a way of switching off the chattering that goes on in our minds when we are preoccupied and under pressure; most of us know how draining and exhausting anxious thoughts can be during times of great stress and tension. However ambitious this might sound, the actual techniques used in meditation are often disarmingly simple: what can be challenging at first is finding the discipline within ourselves to apply the technique.

It is best to sit or lie flat to meditate. Some people choose to sit cross-legged or in a kneeling position, but anyone who feels any discomfort in their spine or knees should avoid these. Sitting in a comfortable, firm-backed chair that allows your feet to make contact with the floor is fine. If you decide to lie down, make sure that your chosen surface is firm, warm and draught-free.

When you are lying down it is best to adopt the position known in yoga as 'the corpse'. This simple posture involves lying in a relaxed way, the arms resting slightly away from the sides of the body, with the backs of the hands making contact with the floor and the palms uppermost. The legs should also fall naturally – slightly apart, with feet loose and relaxed. The back should not be arched, so that the spine and back muscles can completely relax.

Those who prefer to meditate in an upright pose may find it helpful to focus the gaze on something: a flower, a lighted candle or a crystal, or anything else that you feel instinctively is likely to help you reach a meditative state. Focus on the object, putting any other thoughts to one side as they enter the mind (and they will, with a vengeance, as you begin to meditate). As you concentrate on the object, observe what is happening to the pattern of your breathing. Gently regulate it, so that it takes on a steady rhythm, with the in-breath being equal to the out-breath. Others may choose instead to close their eyes and focus on a simple, mentally generated image (the ideal option if you are lying down with your eyes shut).

You may find it helpful to repeat to yourself the simple sound of a single syllable as you breathe in and out. It need be nothing more mystical than repeating the word 'one'; it could be any sound that feels conducive to your quest for a meditative state.

right FOCUSING YOUR GAZE ON AN OBJECT SUCH AS A CANDLE FLAME OR A FLOWER CAN BE AN EFFECTIVE AID TO MEDITATION. below A NEWCOMER TO MEDITATION MIGHT FIND 'THE CORPSE' POSITION FROM YOGA HELPFUL, AS IT ALLOWS THE HEAD, SHOULDERS, ARMS AND LEGS TO RELAX FULLY.

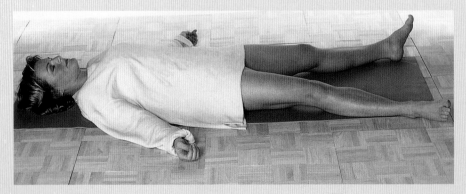

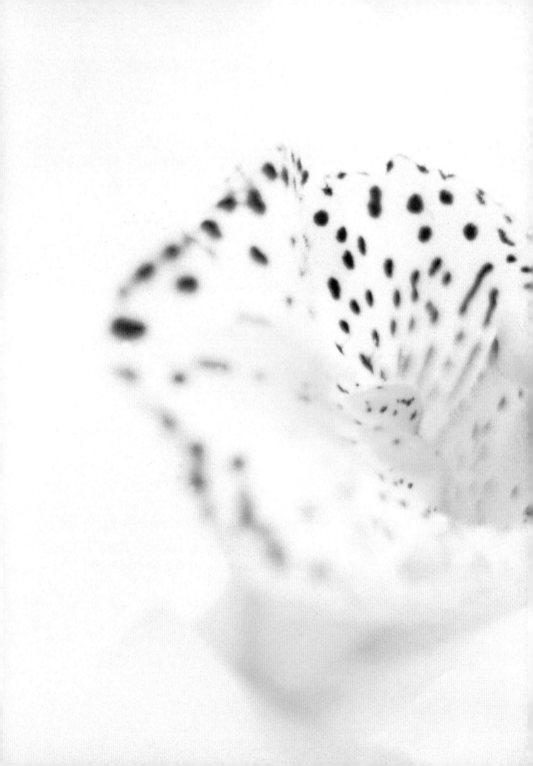

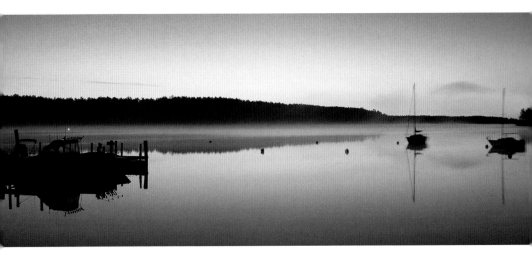

It is important never to rush off at the end of a meditation session; you need to give the mind and body time slowly to engage in regular activity again. When you are ready, open your eyes, stretch your arms and legs, and get up slowly. Above all, if you are lying down, never get up quickly into an upright position: always turn on to your side, and take time to get used to the different sensations in your body as you move to an upright position.

Creative Visualization

This highly pleasurable technique involves taking a mental holiday: focusing the mind on images, sounds and sensations that you associate with somewhere that you feel especially positive about. You should prepare for practising creative visualization in a way similar to that suggested previously for meditation.

Once you are aware that your breathing is steady and regular, call to mind the image of a place that you find relaxing, beautiful or inspiring: it could be somewhere you have actually visited, or an idealized place based on a photograph or a painting. The most important thing is that this should be a place with which you feel you have a very particular rapport.

above CREATIVE VISUALIZATION IS RATHER LIKE TAKING A MENTAL BREAK – 'AWAY FROM IT ALL'.

It does not matter whether it is a peaceful woodland, seashore or pastoral scene, but it must be an environment with which you feel a special connection. As mentally you enter the scene, you will begin to be aware of all the sights, sounds and sensations that are part of this setting. You may choose to lie down and experience the sense of deep relaxation that floods over your body in this enchanted place, or you may continue to walk, slowly discovering new aspects of the scene that draw you further into an even deeper state of relaxation.

You can usefully employ creative visualization in conjunction with progressive muscular relaxation to beneficial effect. Once your muscles are fully relaxed and soft, you can turn your attention to your breathing. As you breathe in, you could choose to see your body being filled with a warm, golden liquid that symbolizes a profound sense of peace, wellbeing and tranquillity. As you breathe out, you can envisage tension, cares and nagging worries leaving the body in a cloud of vapour. Choose whatever colours you feel will give you a sense of personal connection with what you envisage.

Guided Relaxation

As you begin to learn the art of relaxation it can be immensely helpful to use one of the many guided relaxation exercises that are available on tape or CD. This can be especially helpful if you want simply to close your eyes and be taken through a structured relaxation exercise without the pressure of having to decide how to move from one part of the body to another.

Alternatively, you may have found an excellent relaxation exercise described in a book. In this case, it will probably help to record the instructions on a cassette tape or CD. Using your own voice can be a wise strategy, as you may find some of the voices on prerecorded tapes either jarring or monotonous. The following guided exercise is a basic introduction to relaxation. Before you start, prepare yourself according to the guidelines given previously for meditation.

1 Lie on the floor with your knees bent, and your feet roughly 30 cm (12 in) apart. Relax. With one hand resting gently on your belly around the area of your navel, breathe steadily and deeply: your hand should rise and fall with the regular movement of your breath.

2 Listen to your body, and let your breathing pattern follow its own natural pace; never force the rhythm of your breathing. All you need to do at first is to draw your attention to the way you are breathing and observe it.

3 Once your breathing is regular and relaxed, let your legs relax to the floor and adopt the corpse pose described on page 34.

4 Concentrate on the muscles of your head and face. Beginning at the crown of your head, visualize letting go of any tension that is being held in the scalp muscles. Move steadily down your forehead, noting any tension that you encounter on your way. Consciously release any knots of tension and relax each group of muscles before moving on.

5 Move down your body in your mind, stopping wherever there is obvious tension. The jaw, neck, throat, shoulders, hands and lower back are all common areas of muscle tension. Mentally travel to each part of the body in turn, only moving on when each area feels fully relaxed and softened.

6 Once you become familiar with the effect of this process, you should experience a wondrous sense of relaxation and comfort. You may feel as though your body has become much heavier and seems to be sinking through the floor, but it is also common to feel as though your body is so light that it seems to be floating above the surface on which you are lying.

7 Once you feel fully relaxed, turn your attention once again to the pattern of your breathing. You should find that by now it has slowed down and regulated itself to a steady, unforced, relaxed rhythm.

8 As you inhale, visualize yourself being filled with positive energy. As you breathe out, picture any negativity and tension being drawn out of your body. You may choose to use images or colours that have a particular resonance for you, to symbolize positive and negative energy. As time goes on you might feel that you want to change these colours: feel free to make adjustments to match your mood.

9 Luxuriate in this relaxed state for as long as you wish, but make sure that you allow enough time to emerge slowly from the experience of deep relaxation. Rushing back to full activity too quickly can diminish the benefits you will have gained.

10 When you feel ready, start by slowly bringing your attention back to your surroundings. Gently move your head, arms, hands, legs and feet in turn, increasing the size of the movement slowly and steadily until you are making larger flexing and stretching movements. Finally, enjoy a big catlike stretch and open your eyes.

11 Most important of all, never jump up into an upright position after relaxation, but roll on to one side, and spend a little time in a sitting position before finally standing. This is the most effective way of avoiding the light-headedness or feelings of disorientation that may result from getting up too quickly.

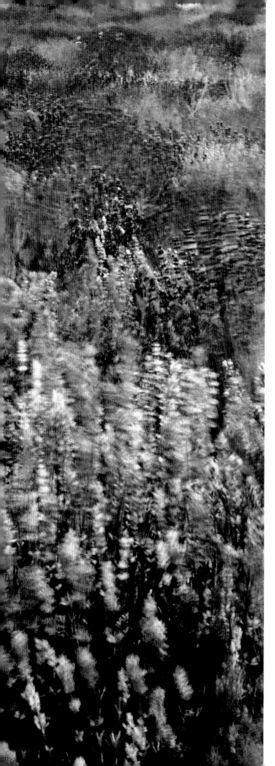

Short-Term Quick Fixes

Here are some rapid-response relaxation techniques to use whenever we feel that tension is building within us. They will quickly induce a state of calm with the minimum amount of fuss.

BREATHE

Stop for a moment and consciously take a few steady, deep breaths that fill your lungs from the base to the tip. This clears the mind, relaxes tension and creates precious time within which consciously to relax.

INHALE

Put a few drops of essential oil of lavender on a tissue and take a whiff if you are feeling uptight and tense.

REFRESH

Use a simple technique called 'palming' to refresh and ease tense, tired eyes: cup your hands and place them over your closed eyes, applying comfortable but firm pressure to the sockets for a few seconds (see page 42).

RELAX

Release all the tension in the neck and shoulders by consciously releasing clenched jaw muscles and letting your shoulders drop significantly as this tension melts away. If you have trouble relaxing the area around your lower jaw, gently press the tip of your tongue against the roof of your mouth just behind your top teeth. This also relaxes the muscles around the temples, thereby discouraging tension headaches.

SMILE

The facial muscles are a primary seat of tension, made manifest in permanent frowning. This will, in turn, contribute to tension headaches and the formation of 'worry lines', which are far from conducive to a sense of wellbeing. The next time you become aware that tension is building, think of something positive, and smile, letting your facial muscles soften.

left LAVENDER IS RENOWNED FOR ITS CALMING AND SEDATIVE PROPERTIES. INHALE THE ESSENTIAL OIL AND PLACE SOME OF THE FRAGRANT FLOWERS IN A SACHET UNDER YOUR PILLOW.

De-stressing at Work

The workplace is a prime suspect for raised stress levels because there are so many factors that are beyond our control. Rumours of decisions to downsize the workforce; the increased pressure of tight deadlines; rapid changes being made in personnel; and the acknowledged health hazards that are a reality in any modern, open-plan, centrally heated and air-conditioned office are just a few of the facts of life at work that can raise our negative stress levels.

As our working environment is such a honey-trap for stress, it makes a great deal of sense to spend some time considering practical steps that we might take to deal effectively with an excess of pressure at work. By taking control in this way, we will be tackling one of the basic factors that can aggravate our general stress levels: feeling powerless about knowing where to begin on the path of stress management.

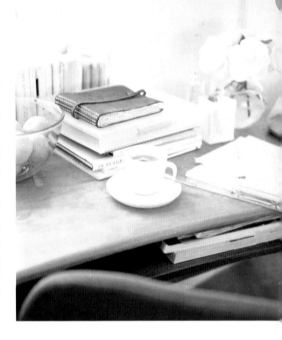

External Factors

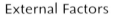 above 'CLUTTER CLEARING' CAN HAVE A HUGELY BENEFICIAL STRESS-REDUCING EFFECT IN THE WORKPLACE.

ORGANIZE

If we feel stressed to the hilt, it can be immensely illuminating and helpful to stop for a moment and consider our surroundings. If we are besieged by a jumble of books, papers and unanswered mail – and this applies to what we see on our computer screens, too – we will, by this general situation unconsciously be reinforcing our feelings of stress and anxiety. If, however, we deliberately take some time to organize our workspace, throwing away anything that is no longer relevant, filing those items that are, and shelving away material that has been building up for months, the benefits will be enormous. We will experience a great psychological lift; feel we have more space in which to work; and be able to locate important material in half the time and with a fraction of the customary frustration and effort.

DELEGATE

Once we learn the art of keeping our workload within manageable boundaries, we will be able to let go of any tasks that can as efficiently and effectively be done by someone else. If we no longer feel that we have to control every piece of work that is presented to us, we are far more likely to make a success of the work with which we are directly involved.

PRIORITIZE

This is really the foundation of effective delegating, because we need to be able to prioritize effectively in order to decide what work we have to do ourselves, and what can be as effectively dealt with by others. How to set about working out priorities at work is a matter of individual preference, but one of the best techniques is still the simplest: list-making. Writing things down on paper has much the same effect as talking about problems: it gets the issues out of our heads, giving us some psychological distance from them. Important tasks demanding most attention should occupy top positions on the list, while those that are less crucial should appear lower down. It also helps to note whether a job needs to be dealt with straightaway, or whether it can be safely put on the

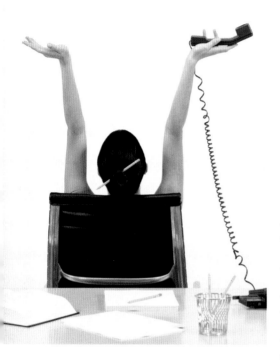

be able to enjoy the pleasure and exhilaration of being stretched and challenged, without having to let some things spill over – to leave us, in the end, feeling overwhelmed. In other words, with a degree of self-knowledge we can keep our commitments within the boundaries of positive stress and avoid letting them drift into the zone of negative stress.

This advice is not offered as a means of avoiding tasks that do not appeal; rather, it is a way of freeing ourselves from unrealistic demands that are causing us a disproportionate amount of stress. When we develop the ability to recognize our limits, we will be well on our way to feeling a great sense of liberation – as well as dealing far more efficiently with those realistic demands with which we are presented. It may also come as a surprise and a relief to discover that we are not in fact as indispensable as we may hitherto have believed.

We may at first find it extremely difficult to take the first step in delegating certain tasks. However, once we get over the initial feelings of uneasiness and unfamiliarity, and become more assertive in managing our workload, we are likely to be delighted by how this delegation can radically reduce our stress levels – surprisingly rapidly, too.

back burner for a little while. Once you have managed to complete a job, make a point of crossing it off the list: it is amazing how therapeutic it can be to see a list like this getting shorter.

EVALUATE

One of the greatest skills of effective time and stress management is one of the most difficult to master at first: the ability to say 'no' to unrealistic demands. Nothing results in quite so much anxiety and stress at work as feeling that we have taken on tasks for which the deadlines appear impossibly tight. In such a situation we need either to be open and frank about not being able to achieve the work in the scheduled time and hand it over, or to negotiate a more realistic timeframe so that we know we can comfortably meet the demands of the project in question.

In order to do this effectively we need to be able realistically to evaluate the maximum workload we can undertake that still allows us to operate effectively and productively. Once we develop this ability we will

ACT

An enormous amount of stress is generated by procrastination, putting off irksome but unavoidable tasks until the very last moment. When we do this, one unfortunate consequence is that we do not forget about the need to deal with the tasks we are constantly postponing. Indeed, they are likely to prey on our minds to an even greater degree, making us feel guilty and uneasy. It is an acknowledged and well-known irony that once we actually get down to a job that we have had 'on hold' for ages, it is usually far less of a chore than we envisaged and we wonder why we loitered so long and did not tackle it sooner.

As taking action is a powerful antidote to negative stress, it stands to reason that postponing action is one of the greatest causes of negative stress. As we shall see, negative emotions, such as anxiety and guilt, play a significant role in raising stress levels. It follows from this that, if we are committed to effective stress management, we should as a priority avoid putting off tasks unnecessarily.

PERSONALIZE

Stand back and take an objective look at your own immediate workspace. If it strikes you as impersonal and drab, this can unwittingly contribute to a lack of inspiration and feelings of stress. Making the effort to make a few minor adjustments is time very well spent, because you are likely to feel uplifted, soothed and energized as a result. Do not overdo it – simply select carefully a few objects about which you feel especially positive: a photograph of a special place, person or pet (or all three combined in one photograph if you are extra lucky!), a small sculpture, a paperweight and a plant, for example. Alternatively, you could choose functional objects – a small selection of self-help books, or an essential-oil vaporizer that could be used to burn stress-reducing or energizing essential oils when you need a boost. Above all, remember to keep it simple: introducing too much will have a cluttering effect, leaving you feeling hemmed-in and stressed.

CLEANSE

Many of us struggle with the pressures of working in an open-plan office, which can be stressful on a number of different levels at once. The cumulative impact of noise can be extremely wearing, as can the lack of privacy if we are having a particularly difficult conversation on the telephone. Toxic chemicals used by fax machines and photocopiers, and exposure to low-grade radiation emitted from VDU screens, are recognized sources of physical stress because they overload our immune systems. If, to this cocktail, we add the problems that come in the wake of poorly functioning air-conditioning and central-heating systems, there is little wonder that many of us feel we

are suffering the ill effects of 'sick building syndrome'. Symptoms can include anything from recurrent tension headaches to persistent infections.

Depressing as this sounds, there are positive steps we can take to minimize the negative effects of working in a modern office. Investing in a desktop ionizer can help guard against feelings of sluggishness and muzzy-headedness, while having plenty of plants around appears to defuse some of the more negative effects of low-grade radiation associated with electrical appliances. If using a custom-made essential-oil burner is not practical at work (not everyone regards the aroma of essential oils as a bonus!), inhaling aromatherapy oils from a tissue can be a simple and invaluable way of clearing the head. Most importantly, go for a walk in the open air at lunchtime rather than just grabbing a sandwich and working

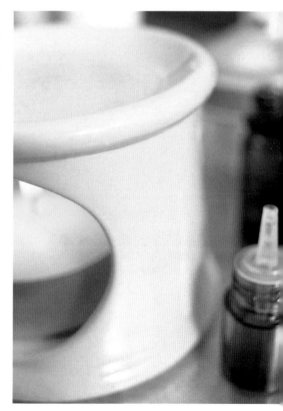

right ESSENTIAL OILS THAT HAVE INVIGORATING OR RELAXING PROPERTIES CAN BE VAPORIZED IN AN OIL BURNER AT HOME OR WORK TO HELP BALANCE OUR MOOD AND ENERGY LEVELS.

through. Not only does this provide a very welcome break from the preoccupations of work, it also forces us to exercise muscles that have probably been inert for an extended period.

Internal Factors

UNWIND

If we work at a desk all day it is easy for physical stress and tension to build up in the neck and shoulders – further aggravated if you are staring at a VDU screen for hours on end. Neck rolls are one of the most effective ways of easing stiffness and tension in the upper body, and they can be done at any time. Lower your head so that your chin rests lightly on your upper chest. Let it roll to the right, letting the natural weight of the head take it back and around to the left-hand side until it comes to rest once again in the centre of your chest. Then repeat the same circular motion, but this time starting with the left and moving to the right.

Shoulder shrugs can also help us to let go of stress and tension, and they work well after neck rolls. Slowly lift up both shoulders towards your ears then drop them down and back. Repeat the motion in reverse by rolling both shoulders back, up towards the ears and down to their original position.

ENERGIZE

Alternate-nostril breathing is an excellent technique used in yoga to clear the mind; it diffuses stress levels and provides a brilliant mental, emotional and physical energy boost when we feel we are flagging. Begin by bending the three middle fingers into the palm of the right hand, keeping the thumb and little finger extended. Rest your thumb gently against your right nostril and breathe through the left nostril for a count of four. Then close both nostrils by putting your little finger on your left nostril, holding your breath for a count of four. Release your thumb and exhale from your right nostril for the same count. Pause for a moment before repeating the cycle, beginning this time with the side you have just breathed out from. If you repeat the process four times on each side you will find your mind is much clearer and more focused.

RELAX

Take some of the strain and tension out of your face by closing your eyes for a moment or two while you consciously rest the jaw, neck and shoulder muscles. 'Palming', as described on page 38, can also help to relax the eyes and facial muscles. If you work for long periods at a VDU screen, or spend hours reading intricate documents, not only do you need to take regular breaks, you must also blink regularly. Staring at a screen for an excessively long time without blinking will strain your eyes, which will become dry and bloodshot. Blinking can also help to prevent the headaches that result from overstressed, tired eyes.

below 'PALMING' IS A TECHNIQUE THAT CAN BE EMPLOYED TO RELAX BOTH THE EYES AND FACIAL MUSCLES.

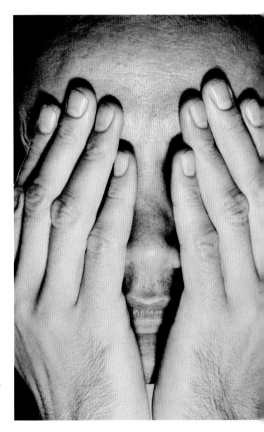

De-stressing at Home

Most of the basic principles behind the de-stress techniques recommended for the workplace can be applied equally well at home if we use a little flair and imagination. Clearing clutter, delegating household chores, prioritizing tasks, organizing our surroundings better, and taking positive action rather than endlessly procrastinating: these are all as relevant to stress management at home as they are at work.

However, there are some additional practical measures that can help us transform our homes into havens where negative stress is more likely to be defused than created.

TRANQUILLITY

We all need a space to which we can retreat when life gets too tough. This is especially true if we are immersed in family pressures as well as professional ones. The combined needs of young children and elderly relatives make a potent mixture, often leaving us with a profound sense that we have little space for ourselves. Although we can create this important space in our minds through the regular use of relaxation and meditation techniques, we also need to find a physical space that we find calming and soothing. Any room in the house can fulfil this function, but one of the easiest rooms to turn into our de-stress sanctuary is the bathroom. After all, unless we have very young children, no one, as a rule, is likely to follow us there. Practical advice on how to turn your bathroom into a stress-proofing sanctuary appears in Chapter Five.

SOUND

Music can be a powerful mood enhancer and stress reliever. Whatever we choose needs to suit our mood and temperament; it should by no means be limited to New Age pieces. Although controversial, it has been suggested in some studies that exposure to unrelieved heavy metal music can induce feelings of negativity and depression in susceptible people. On the other hand, exposure to baroque music appears to have the opposite effect. Of course, this does not mean that we have to avoid rock music and

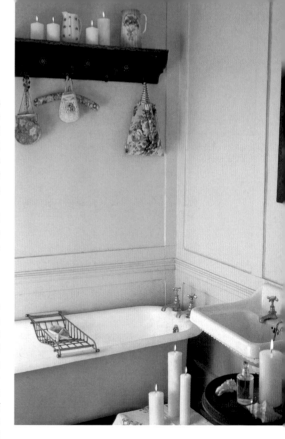

above **THE BATHROOM, MORE THAN MOST OTHER ROOMS IN THE HOME, NATURALLY LENDS ITSELF TO RELAXING ACTIVITIES.**

limit ourselves to listening to classical compositions. We just need to choose music that leaves us feeling emotionally balanced, uplifted and relaxed.

LIGHT

The importance of maximum exposure to natural light in reducing symptoms of depression and anxiety has attracted much attention over the past decade. In a recent British television documentary, which filmed a family attempting to live in a 1940s house for a limited period, the importance of light emerged in a fascinating way. One of the significantly stressful elements of living in the house proved to be the use of blackout curtains, which the modern occupants of the house found extremely depressing and claustrophobic. This brings home to us how much we take for granted the possibilities for generous lighting in modern housing: not until it is removed do we really appreciate its positive effects.

If we live in a house that gets little natural light during the day, we might consider fitting bulbs that mimic natural daylight. Equally, some of us tend to become sad or emotionally flat at night if we feel that a room is unduly dark or gloomy. The strategic placement of light fixtures can do a great deal to create an uplifting effect. On the other hand, however, others might welcome the softness that comes with low-level lighting, finding that it has a distinctly calming effect.

We can buffer the stress of having to wake up early by using a bedside light that mimics the effect of dawning daylight by building slowly in intensity. This can even be combined in some models with recorded birdsong. In the evening, if we are feeling stressed and uptight, we may find it helpful to burn a candle scented with relaxing essential oils, such as lavender or rose.

SCENT

Perfumes and naturally occurring aromas have been shown to have a powerful effect on our mood and state of mind. Many of us will have experienced the mood-enhancing effect of certain smells at first hand if we have unexpectedly caught a whiff of an aroma that powerfully conjures up the memory of a place, person or significant experience. At such a moment, we experience again the emotions connected with the remembered event as though we have been transported back in time. And all as a result of catching a drift of perfume.

As aromas can have an attractive or repellent quality, it makes sense to surround ourselves with those that have a positive effect on us. Our taste is likely to be determined by the mood we happen to be in at any given time, so we need to be prepared to ring the changes accordingly. For instance, if we start the day feeling muzzy-headed and slow, a light

right THE FURNISHINGS AND COLOURS THAT WE CHOOSE WHEN WE ARE DECORATING CAN TURN OUR HOME INTO A STRESS-REDUCING SANCTUARY.

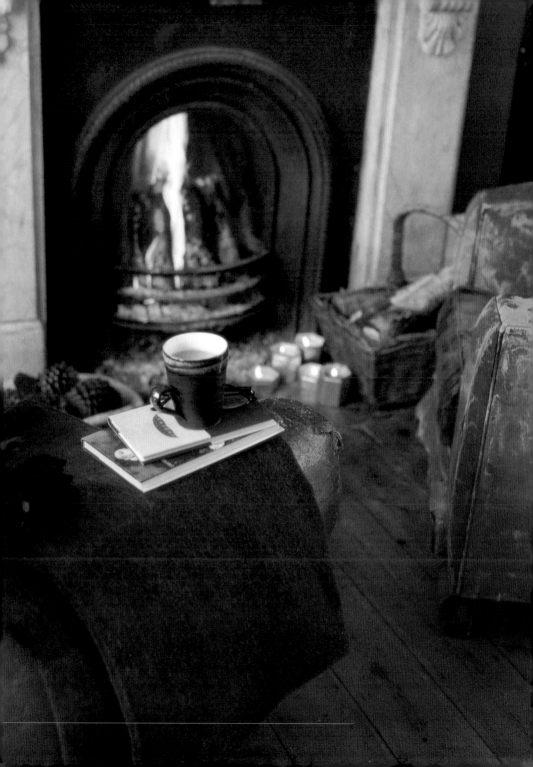

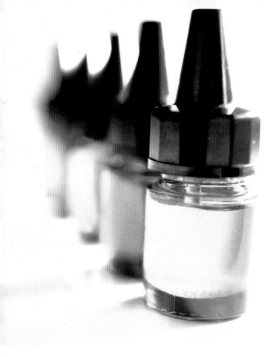

left ESSENTIAL OILS CAN BE ADDED TO A WARM BATH TO MAXIMIZE ITS RELAXING EFFECT. below FOREST COLOURS IN A HOME CAN EVOKE THE SERENITY OF A WOODLAND WALK.

The colour groupings to which we are most attracted say a great deal about our personalities. After all, we make colour choices every day, from the clothes we wear to the more enduring decoration of our homes.

If we feel that we need to create a calming and soothing effect, surrounding ourselves with blue-based tones may be of great benefit. Crimson and orange, in contrast, are thought to be energizing; while yellow is uplifting; and green apparently has the capacity to help balance our moods. As always, we should follow our instincts: whatever choices we make should grow out of our personal preferences. After all, there is little to be gained from surrounding ourselves with various shades of 'mood-balancing' green if we detest the colour.

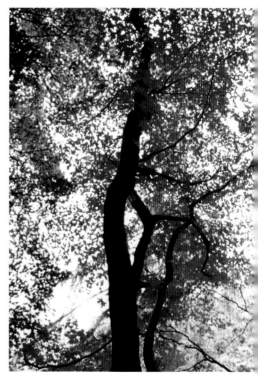

burst of citrus-based essential oils, such as grapefruit, or refreshing peppermint or rosemary, can go a substantial way to energize and revitalize us. Bergamot – another citrus-based oil – is also uplifting. On the other hand, if we are feeling volatile or on an emotional 'short fuse', using mood-balancing oils, such as ylang ylang, geranium or clary sage may be of more benefit. Essential oil of basil, meanwhile, as it is good for concentration, might also be used as a stress-busting aroma; it might help to instil a degree of focus in someone overwhelmed and paralysed – like a rabbit in headlights – by indecision.

There are today vast numbers of shower products and bath oils infused with essential oils, and scented candles as well; or you can burn essential oils in a custom-made vaporizer.

COLOUR

Many of us know instinctively that colour can have a powerful effect on our mood, with certain colours stimulating an upbeat mood that exudes vitality, and others making us feel profoundly tranquil and blissed out. Some colours are sociable while others can be regarded as more contemplative and quiet.

Confronting Negative Demons: How to Avoid Self-Sabotage

We can unwittingly create more stress for ourselves by approaching challenging situations from a negative emotional perspective. Responses such as anxiety, guilt, resentment and unexpressed anger do not give us any support as we try to resolve life's challenges; in fact, they do just the opposite – they actively hold us back from looking at a situation from a balanced emotional perspective.

As a result of the negative imbalance that these emotions bring in their wake, we are likely to find that in a crisis we react in a way that can often make problems more complex and convoluted. If, on the other hand, we develop ways of bringing a more positive mental and emotional focus into play, we will find that solutions present themselves both more easily and more quickly. This, in turn, gives us a feeling of assurance, which supplies the support we need to take further assertive action. Soon we are being swept up in a positive spiral of our own making that can play a centrally important role in reducing negative stress in our lives.

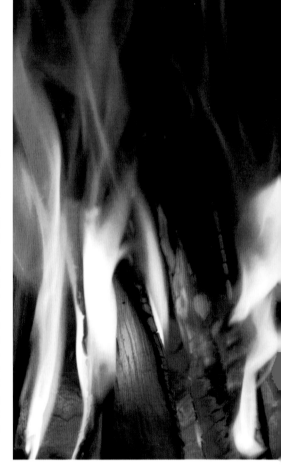

Suppressed Anger

Although some of us may feel uncomfortable with anger as an emotion, it is important to recognize that in its appropriate place, justifiably expressed anger can be a positive, liberating experience. Conversely, if we are constantly repressing anger, or repeatedly losing our temper for very little reason, this can have an extremely negative effect on our personalities. Mismanaged fury can leave us extremely vulnerable to feelings of resentment, bitterness and – eventually – depression, and none of these is empowering in our attempt to deal with negative stress.

If we see ourselves as being on a permanent 'short fuse' at home and at work, there is a very strong chance that we are suppressing a powerful feeling of anger from the past that may be associated with a much more significant, unresolved issue. The next time we are about to fly into a disproportionate rage, it might be very helpful and illuminating to stop and consider what we are really feeling at that moment. The chances are that we will discover that we are completely overreacting to the focus of our anger and irritation. Once we give ourselves time to question why we are reacting so intensely to the immediate problem, we have a much better chance of gaining a possible insight into the roots of our anger. And when we can do this, we are offered an important opportunity to be able justifiably to express our anger in response to the original situation.

above **UNLEASH YOUR FIREY TEMPER: APPROPRIATELY EXPRESSED ANGER CAN BE LIBERATING, BURNING UP GRIEVANCES AND HURTS.**

The secret of healthy anger management lies in learning assertiveness skills rather than being trigger-happily angry. When we adopt an assertive stance, we become empowered to react in an appropriate way to a stressful situation. As a result of this balanced, considered response, the chances that the outcome will be positive are far greater than if we simply lose our temper.

The first rule of assertiveness training is to learn the skill of speaking our minds in a clear, constructive and forceful way. It helps always to remember that an assertive perspective is entirely the opposite of an angry one, because anger prevents us from taking control of a situation and, as a result, we become less rather than more powerful. Once we are flooded with anger we find it impossible to see any situation in a balanced way, and instead we are primed to overreact at the slightest provocation. In addition, being constantly at the mercy of hair-trigger moods is extremely draining. Just consider how exhausting an outburst of anger is, and imagine expending that level of energy regularly.

How to be Assertive

There are three vitally important elements that should be brought into play whenever we are dealing with a situation that demands basic assertiveness skills:

- Assessing the problematic situation as objectively, succinctly and fairly as we can.
- Expressing our feelings as clearly as possible, avoiding the trap of placing unnecessary guilt on another party or taking a heavy-handed, judgmental stance. If there are others involved in the situation, try to sidestep the issue, take a deep breath and avoid losing your temper, then come back calmly and firmly to the point that needs to be made.
- Suggesting a course of action that will result in correcting or positively changing the nature of the problem.

Guilt

This is another of the most negative, inhibiting, stress-inducing emotions that we can suffer, especially if we are punishing ourselves unnecessarily with guilty feelings that are disproportionate to the reality of the situation. It often helps to look to the past to see whether the roots of our tendency to suffer from unwarranted guilt were unwittingly instilled in us during childhood.

Remember how we were treated by parents, siblings, friends or lovers. Were we made to feel valued, gifted and special, or have we been left with an abiding sense of feeling overlooked, criticized and undervalued? Unfortunately, if we have felt that we never quite reached the standards set for us by others, there is a strong possibility that we will still unwittingly be striving for an unrealistic standard of perfection in order to earn the love and positive attention that we are craving. In truth, no one is perfect, so we are bound to fall painfully short of the standards that we keep on trying to achieve. And when evidence of this begins to emerge, we are preprogrammed to respond by feeling painful emotions of guilt and inadequacy.

If we are to move on positively, we need to break out of this negative, self-punishing cycle, liberating ourselves from emotional patterns that by now fit us like a second skin. This will certainly be painful in the early stages, but once we become familiar with the new sensations that will emerge as a result of our challenging deeply ingrained preconceptions of ourselves, we will be very reluctant to return to our habitual ways of reacting.

If we find that our feelings of guilt are especially resistant to change, we may need professional guidance and support in order to move on. Seeking help, and not feeling guilty about doing so, is an important first step. The sort of constructive support that is appropriate in this case may be obtained from a cognitive behavioural therapist, whose training enables him or her to encourage clients to identify for themselves certain ingrained patterns of emotional behaviour. Once we know how these patterns work, we are free to react differently if we so choose.

Controlling Guilt

Resisting unfair and unrealistic feelings of guilt involves taking the following practical steps:

- The next time you feel haunted by guilty feelings, try to stand back mentally from the situation and assess as fairly as possible how merited these feelings are. There is a good chance that you will have done the best you could in a difficult situation. On the other hand, you may, with the benefit of hindsight, feel that you could have acted differently, and so will decide to use this insight if and when you are in a similar situation in the future.

- If feelings of guilt are focused on a particular issue or individual, it can be very helpful to look more closely at this situation. We may feel, on reflection, that we could take more positive action in order to come closer to resolving the situation, but equally it may become obvious that we really are doing as much as we possibly can to move the situation in a more positive direction, but that we are not getting the vital cooperation we need from others to be successful. If this latter is true, we may need mentally to let go of the situation, or even to consider staying away from people or situations that induce unfair feelings of guilt.

- Aim to consciously boost your confidence levels by celebrating your positive qualities. Should someone pay you a compliment, accept it at face value rather than searching for a negative motive behind it. When things are going well in your life, try to lose yourself in the pleasure of the moment and bask for a while. And, most important of all, it is essential that you discard any underlying belief in the adage that laughter will be followed by tears.

right LETTING GO OF ANY NEGATIVE FEELINGS WE MAY HAVE BEEN CARRYING AROUND FROM THE PAST LEAVES US FREE TO ENJOY THE PRESENT.

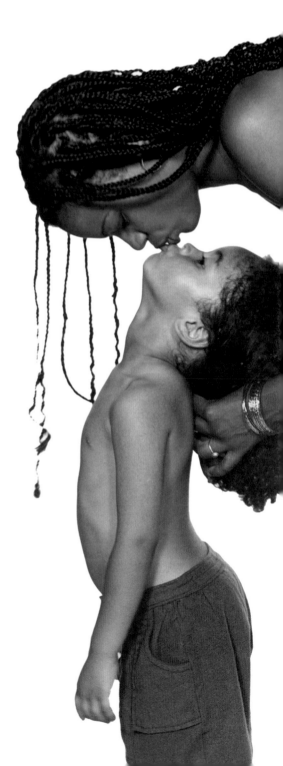

Fear

Frequently feeling fearful is extraordinarily stressful. As we have already seen, constantly triggering the fight-or-flight response leaves us feeling exhausted, indecisive and unable to function in a focused, productive way. Unreasonable fear holds us back from enjoying life in so many ways: chronic lack of confidence can prevent us from developing relationships and stifle professional advancement; irrational phobias can prevent us from enjoying basic pleasures, such as travelling and socializing, or facing life's basic challenges; and a disproportionate fear of ageing can prevent us from enjoying the present.

Some fears that seem huge are, in reality, quite manageable. Public speaking, for instance, may be a petrifying prospect, but even if you never relish being the centre of attention, you will – if you build up your confidence slowly and steadily – gradually boost your self-esteem and basic confidence if you make yourself stand up and speak.

The roots of free-floating fear frequently lie in our upbringing. Sadly, many of us may have had fearful reactions unwittingly instilled in us as children, when parents may have used phrases such as 'the bogey man will get you if you don't stop . . .' to discipline us. Statements like this repeated to children at a formative stage can have the very negative effect of making them see the world as a dangerous and frightening place where, if they do not behave well, something nasty will happen to them.

Fear can also be communicated subconsciously to a young child by a parent who is chronically fearful and anxious. There is a very strong chance that a parent who finds the world a threatening place may hand this conviction on to his or her children, unless positive steps are taken to prevent this.

Some of us may also have suffered traumatic experiences at an impressionable age. Witnessing a serious accident, sexual abuse, or some such violent episode are likely to leave mental and emotional scars that can make us fearful and insecure as adults.

right FEAR CAN FREEZE US TO SUCH AN EXTENT THAT WE ARE UNABLE TO ENJOY WARM RELATIONSHIPS.

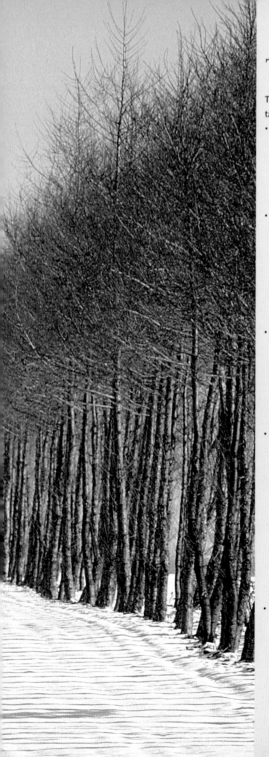

Taming Fear

There are positive steps that we can take to tame unreasonable fear:

- If specific phobias are limiting our lives in an unreasonable way, it is worth seeking professional help and support, such as behavioural therapy. Relaxation techniques using controlled breathing can also be combined with behavioural therapy.
- Creative visualization techniques can play an important role in helping us disperse anxious feelings, too. If we picture a situation where we would normally feel threatened, it can be very helpful to conjure up a positive version of this same image, transforming the outcome into a positive one – by deliberately changing the negative imagery.
- Those of us who battle with feelings of ongoing anxiety linked to a lack of self-esteem may benefit a great deal from reading some of the many self-help books available on building self-confidence. Consult the Recommended Reading section at the back of this book (see page 124) for details of some of these titles.
- If irrational fears have been instilled in us from childhood, we may benefit greatly from cognitive therapy. Working with a cognitive therapist we are encouraged to identify negative patterns of behaviour that are so familiar to our perspective on life that we are quite unaware that they exist. Once these habitual thought patterns have been identified, we have the ability to break free from them. The therapist can show us ways to shed these negative emotional habits from the past and move on without them.
- By confronting situations that make us feel irrationally fearful or nervous we can liberate ourselves from the tyranny of anxiety. We should always build up our confidence slowly but surely by taking small steps, which will enable us to build up our confidence as we proceed. This avoids the risk of taking on too much and regretting having made the attempt.

Getting Personal: Intimate Relationships

Many of us may already be aware of the way that feeling overly stressed for too long very often makes us use the very people we are closest to as punchbags. Too many pressures at work and at home will often make us either irritable with our partners or withdrawn, which, if we are not careful, will lead to a further downward spiral laden with negative stress.

If these issues are not addressed, our physical relationship is unlikely to thrive and develop. Trouble and strife in the bedroom only makes the situation worse, as a disappointing sex life simply introduces further stress. Enjoying any sensual pleasure to the full depends fundamentally on a sense of relaxation, so problems such as impotence and diminished sexual arousal – acknowledged stress-related problems – will only pile on the pressure when it is least needed.

Alternative and complementary therapists are very aware that a significantly high percentage of the patients consulting them for a range of stress-related problems will confess to having abysmally low energy levels – mental, emotional and physical – and a therapist can more or less guarantee that if a patient is exhausted in this way, libido will also be flat. It is not unusual for a patient to admit that there are times when a stiff drink or even just a cup of tea is a more attractive proposition than a passionate encounter.

There is good news. The situation can often be effectively reversed, because as soon as energy levels improve, a sense of 'get up and go' is re-established, and stress-reduction techniques are brought into play. It is also important to bear in mind that a regular, enthusiastic and balanced sex life has been shown to bring with it a host of benefits – apart from the obvious one – including increased immune system performance and a decrease in stress-related symptoms. The most crucial thing to remember is the need for vigilance (essential if the situation is not to slide further and further down an unsatisfactory, slippery slope) and preventative action. Here are some basic suggestions that should help to revitalize a flagging relationship:

TALK

Almost all relationship breakdowns are caused by a lack of communication of one sort or another. Not having enough time to talk through important issues can widen an emotional gulf between partners. If this happens, fairly trivial matters can begin to grow into much larger issues that become much harder to deal with, and which, unfortunately, are likely to be put on hold for even longer, further compounding the problem. The trick is to make time together a definite priority: making a conscious effort to relax together with a drink at the end of the day, for example, rather than automatically lounging in front of the television or surfing the Internet.

TIME ALONE

One of the most difficult aspects of having a young family is having time for each other, especially when both partners are working, because often, by the time their children are in bed, all they are fit for themselves is to fall into bed and (if lucky) go to sleep. One of the best ways to restore the passion to a relationship suffering from the demands of young children is to arrange to have child-free weekend breaks at regular intervals. This makes possible the spontaneity that is a necessary cornerstone of keeping a relationship alive.

GOING WITH THE FLOW

Be aware of your body clock and avoid the temptation to make love at the end of the day purely as a matter of habit or tradition. Some of us may find that this suits the natural rhythm of our libido, but others may find the afternoon more arousing. The logistics of this may require a little ingenuity but it is well worth the effort. Think of the French! Think of the Italians! What did you imagine the siesta was for?

TOUCH

It is sometimes too easy in a long-term relationship to forget to touch each other, except when it is going to lead to lovemaking. A hug, holding hands and putting an arm around a partner are all valuable ways of maintaining physical intimacy and communicating – at the most basic level.

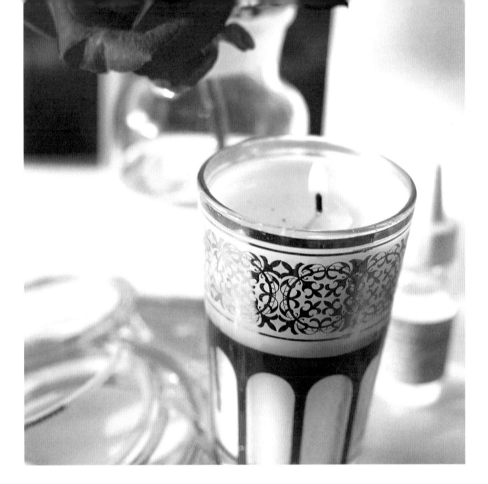

HUMOUR

A sense of humour can be a very sexy attribute in a partner, as spontaneous laughter can go a long way towards establishing a close connection. While laughter at an inappropriate moment can be a passion killer, if it is expressed opportunely it can also be an excellent stress-diffuser. After all, if sex were always deadly serious it would become very dull indeed.

SCENE-SETTING

Bedrooms need to be sensual places where we can delight in the sensations of touch, smell and sight. We can be as imaginative with décor as we please, but we should include soft, diffused lighting, and fabrics that are sensually pleasing. In addition, an essential oil such as ylang ylang, jasmine or sandalwood can be

above **WITH A LITTLE IMAGINATION OUR BEDROOM CAN EASILY BE TRANSFORMED INTO THE PERFECT PLACE FOR A ROMANTIC ENCOUNTER.**

vaporized as a stress-reliever and mood enhancer – or used in massage oils and rubbed in gently (though those with sensitive skins should forgo this).

MOOD FOOD

There are a variety of foods and spices that are reputed to have aphrodisiac properties, so you might like to include some, or all, of them in your diet when libido has taken a nosedive – and even if it has not. Asparagus, shellfish, celery, parsnips, ginger and cinnamon are all ingredients that are credited with boosting libido.

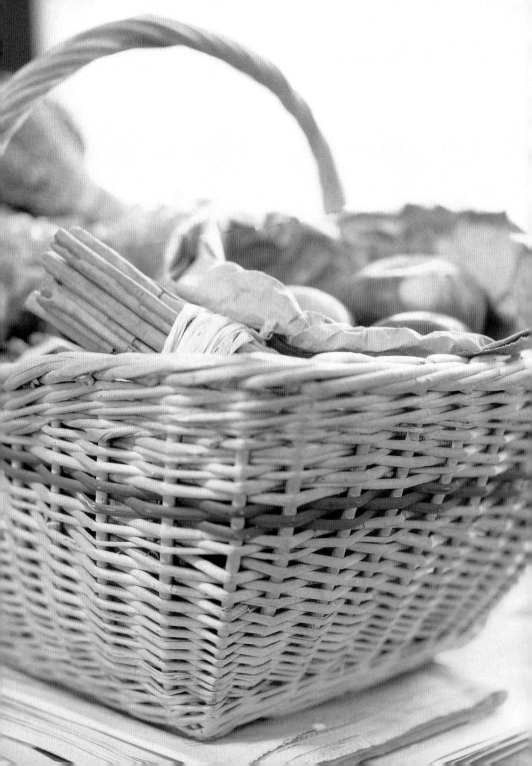

4 Nourish: The Nutritional Stress-Proofing Plan

THE INTIMATE CONNECTION BETWEEN WHAT WE EAT AND DRINK AND THE QUALITY OF MENTAL AND EMOTIONAL BALANCE THAT WE ENJOY IS INCREASINGLY ACKNOWLEDGED BY NUTRITION EXPERTS. ANYONE WHO HAS EXPERIENCED THE TEMPORARY HIGH THAT COMES FROM EATING CHOCOLATE, OR KNOWS THE 'WIRED-UP', JITTERY FEELING THAT COMES AFTER A COUPLE OF CUPS OF ESPRESSO COFFEE IN QUICK SUCCESSION KNOWS THAT CERTAIN FOODS AND DRINKS CAN HAVE DRAMATIC EFFECTS ON OUR BODIES.

What we may not have appreciated, however, is that the sense of fatigue or irritability that follows in a comparatively short period of time will also be connected; it is an after-effect of these items. This is partly because of the chemical imbalance that results from the stimulation of coffee's hefty dose of caffeine and from exposure to the feelgood chemicals contained in chocolate: acknowledged to be addictive substances, they both leave the body craving for more within a relatively short space of time. Ironically, they are also the very props we are instinctively tempted to turn to in times of negative stress and pressure.

In addition, both coffee and chocolate wreak a destabilizing effect on our blood-sugar levels. This chapter will explain how important it is to maintain

left BLOOD-SUGAR LEVELS RESPOND MORE POSITIVELY TO WHOLEMEAL, UNREFINED GRAINS THAN TO WHITE, PROCESSED PRODUCTS, MADE FROM REFINED INGREDIENTS.

stable blood-sugar levels if we are to enjoy maximum vitality, and mental and emotional well-being; and how crucial a role the regulation of blood-sugar levels can play in keeping stress-related problems at bay. In many ways, healthy blood-sugar levels provide the vital key to our being able to take whatever punches life may throw at us.

This is also where we gain a working knowledge of how to discard the foods and drinks that intensify our negative stress load, while learning to identify the dietary ingredients that can calm and soothe our minds, emotions and bodies.

Do not worry if all this sounds tough and spartan. The advice that follows has been compiled with a full awareness that eating and drinking is often as much about delighting the senses as it is about nourishing the body. As a result, recommendations have been designed to allow us to create a varied, flexible and delicious eating plan that is highly unlikely to leave us feeling deprived or limited as regards choice.

Most importantly, the dietary suggestions that follow can easily be applied by those of us with a demanding, stressful lifestyle. High-powered jobs that give us little time for food preparation; varied and numerous family demands; the need occasionally to fall back on ready-made meals; and the basic human desire for an occasional treat: all these have been taken into account. Bon appetit!

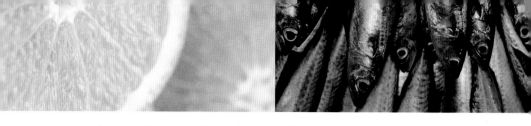

Foods and Drinks that Alleviate Stress

PROTEIN FOODS
Fish, chicken, or pulses
combined with cereal

Eaten in small quantities regularly, these stimulate the production of
dopamine in the body, which can be converted to adrenaline in times
of stress, providing us with an extra 'edge'.

COMPLEX CARBOHYDRATES
Including brown rice,
potatoes and wholegrain
products, such as bread,
pasta and cereals

We should always choose these rather than their refined relatives when
we are under pressure. Complex carbohydrates are broken down in the
body at a pace that promotes a sustained release of energy, whereas
refined carbohydrates provide us with an initial sugar 'rush' that very
quickly leaves us muzzy-headed, grouchy and exhausted.

'B-RICH' FOODS
Foods that are a rich source
of vitamin B complex

The B complex vitamin group plays a major role in supporting our
nervous system in times of maximum stress. Brewer's yeast, dairy
foods, wholegrains, green, leafy vegetables and seafood are all B rich.

BANANAS

A prime source of the natural antidepressant amino acid tryptophan.

**AVOCADOS, ORANGES,
DAIRY FOODS AND LETTUCE**

Generally regarded as foods with a sedative effect, these help us
to unwind when we are feeling short-fused. This may be because
they contain bromine, which acts on the body as a natural relaxant.

CAMOMILE TEA

One of the most soothing, calming beverages available. This should be
the drink of choice at bedtime because it has a sleep-inducing effect. If
we are really stressed and finding it difficult to sleep, it will help to soak
in a warm bath scented with a strong infusion of camomile flowers: drop
a few camomile teabags under the hot tap (faucet) while the bath is running.

**FRESHLY SQUEEZED FRUIT
AND VEGETABLE JUICES**

Juices made from yellow, orange, dark green or red fruit and vegetables
are a rich source of antioxidant nutrients, which have been shown to play
a pivotal role in supporting our immune systems at times of stress.

**LIBERAL QUANTITIES OF
MINERAL OR FRESHLY
FILTERED WATER**

Many of us are moderately dehydrated most of the time. We need
to drink at least five large glasses of water each day. Symptoms of low-
grade dehydration often resemble those of stress-related problems –
headaches, constipation and skin problems, for example.

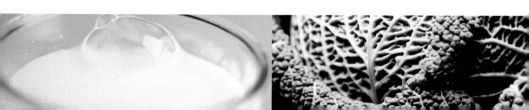

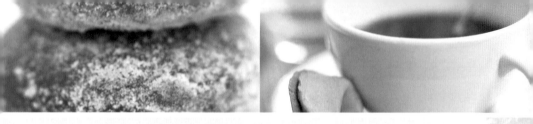

Foods and Drinks that Aggravate Stress

CONVENIENCE FOODS
High in chemical preservatives, flavourings and colourings

When eaten regularly, these foods can place a heavy toxic burden on the body. Some commonly found additives, such as monosodium glutamate (MSG), can contribute to stress-related headaches and intensify allergic symptoms.

FOODS AND DRINKS HIGH IN REFINED SUGAR
Cakes, cookies, fizzy drinks and sweets

Refined (white) sugar is known to trigger erratic energy levels and contribute to fatigue and lowered performance of the immune system. Common reactions to an excess of sugar include poor concentration and light-headedness.

COFFEE, TEA AND CAFFEINATED SOFT DRINKS

Caffeine is a drug that should be treated with caution at all times; it is highly addictive in nature and can trigger insomnia, jitteriness and irritability. Moreover, caffeine withdrawal tends to cause severe headaches, often accompanied by light-headedness and queasiness. Tea contains slightly less caffeine than coffee but enough to cause the same problems when drunk regularly. All caffeinated drinks have the same properties – to a greater or lesser degree.

CHOCOLATE

Eating quantities of delicious and apparently comforting chocolate too often will lead to problems similar to those of caffeine addiction, as chocolate combines sugar and caffeine among its basic ingredients.

ALCOHOL

Although alcohol helps us to relax initially, a long-term high intake will trigger sleep disturbance, digestive problems, headaches, mood swings and poor levels of concentration. Alcohol also places a toxic burden on our immune systems.

CIGARETTES

Cigarettes can have a fairly immediate effect, making us feel mellower or more alert, but even marginal withdrawal from nicotine triggers irritability, poor concentration and an increase in appetite. There is solid evidence to suggest that the long-term effects of smoking mimic those of the stress response, and smoking cigarettes regularly – in whatever quantity – is known to put us at increased risk of developing stress-related conditions, such as heart disease.

Eating to De-stress

Here the basic nutritional boundaries we should aim to work within are explained. Inevitably, there will be occasions when this is easier to do than at others, but whatever happens, do not get stressed about it. Stay within this basic framework on a day-to-day basis, and the odd occasion when you stray beyond will do no major or lasting damage.

If you follow this basic advice you will soon find that you not only deal with the stresses of daily life more resiliently, but also reap important benefits in your general vitality and overall health. Those common stress-related headaches, recurrent minor infections and digestive problems should become a dim and distant memory.

Variety

In order to guard against boredom, make sure that meals do not become monotonous: try to vary your eating patterns according to the dictates of your tastebuds.

If you are a meat-eater, try to cut down dramatically on red meat in favour of poultry or turkey. Also ring the changes by treating yourself to a meat-free high-protein meal at least once a week: a casserole or curry made from pulses and beans combined with brown rice, for example.

Generally, avoid rich puddings for at least four days a week, choosing fresh fruit and bio yogurt instead. Have one glass of wine of your choice, if you wish, and plenty of mineral water. A warming cup of camomile tea before bed can help to relax the mind and induce a sound sleep.

Remember that it will not help you to stick rigorously to the advice above if to do so would cause you stress. You may need sometimes to swap lunch with dinner if you are having a business lunch, or you may find you want your cup of real coffee mid-morning rather than mid-afternoon.

right ALWAYS MAKE A POINT OF HAVING BREAKFAST, OTHERWISE YOU ARE LIKELY TO BE HIT HARD BY A SLUMP IN ENERGY LEVELS BY MID-MORNING.

Stress–Free Eating Plan

BREAKFAST
Your first meal of the day should consist of complex carbohydrates in the form of cereal with semi-skimmed milk and wholemeal toast with a little butter, preserve or honey. Fresh fruit will provide important fibre as well as antioxidant nutrients (freshly squeezed juice will give nutrients, but not the fibre). In the winter you may also like to have the occasional free-range poached or scrambled egg on wholemeal toast. Try free-range duck eggs for a richer taste and firmer texture.

MID-MORNING
A piece of fruit and a cup of fruit or herbal tea will supply an energy boost. Alternatively, have another glass of freshly squeezed fruit and/or vegetable juice.

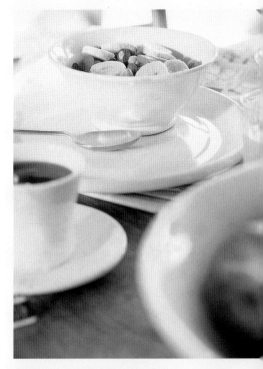

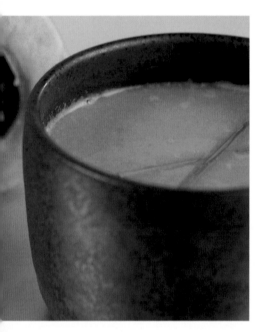

DINNER

Your evening meal can be as varied as you want to make it. Choose any variety of fish (poached and dressed) and eat it with a huge salad in summer or with generous helpings of dark green, orange and red vegetables in winter, plus potatoes or brown rice. Choose an oily fish (mackerel, salmon or fresh sardines) for major health benefits or opt for cod, tuna, trout or swordfish. Poultry in the form of chicken or turkey can make a change, but try – if at all possible – to buy a bird that has been reared free range. A large dish of pasta topped with a sauce of your choice and a sprinkling of ground pinenuts, sesame seeds or croutons would be a good alternative, especially for vegetarians.

left HOME-MADE SOUP IS A QUICK BUT NOURISHING LUNCH.
below BE IMAGINATIVE IN YOUR CHOICE OF VEGETABLES AND IN THE WAY YOU COOK THEM.

LUNCH

The midday meal can consist of either a large salad or roasted vegetables with couscous, or a baked potato. A mixed salad sandwich on wholemeal bread could be a lighter alternative, while in winter a bowl of chunky vegetable soup with beans and pulses added might be more appealing. Drink a large glass or two of water at lunchtime, with or a twist of lemon or lime or some natural fruit flavouring added.

MID-AFTERNOON

Energy is likely to slump during the afternoon, but a cup of green tea (full of antioxidants but naturally low in caffeine) and a handful of dried fruit and fresh nuts (ideally brazils, walnuts or almonds, which are a rich source of essential fatty acids) will kickstart your batteries. If green tea does not appeal, try one of the many coffee substitutes on the market or, if you really are desperate for a cup of the real stuff, have one weak cafe latte – and resolve to not let it become a custom.

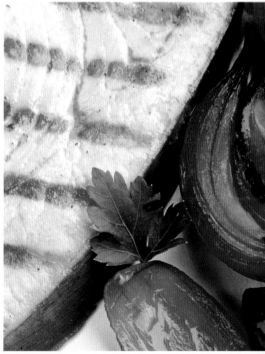

Kicking the Sugar Habit

Too much sugar has the undesirable effect of causing rollercoaster energy levels, while also contributing to erratic mood swings and diminished levels of concentration – a catalogue of negative effects, before you have even considered the additional physical problems that result from too high a consumption of refined sugar: obesity, dental cavities and an increased predisposition to diabetes.

Try to avoid adding refined sugar to hot drinks. Ideally, try to take them unsweetened, but you could add a little raw honey to start with. Once you get used to the unsweetened flavour, you will quickly wonder why you ever added sugar. Cut down on sticky cakes and cookies with high levels of refined sugar, choosing pieces of fresh fruit or organic savoury rice cakes instead. If sugar cravings do not go away, have an occasional organic, oat-based cookie.

It is important to avoid 'diet' or 'low-calorie' versions of anything – fizzy drinks, snacks, puddings, cookies or yogurts. 'Diet' may mean less sugar, but these products will be packed with chemical artificial sweeteners that we can well do without.

Not only do artificial sweeteners, such as saccharin, leave a most unpleasant, bitter aftertaste in the mouth; the full extent of the health problems that may arise from a regular intake of these chemical additives is not yet known. One of the most commonly used sweeteners (aspartame) has already been shown to exacerbate the stress response by triggering stimulation of the brain, while long-term use appears adversely to affect levels of serotonin (the much talked-about, feelgood neurotransmitter), aggravating depression. Sorbitol, meanwhile, when taken in regular or generous doses is also known to cause noticeable gastric upsets, such as diarrhoea.

It is salutary to carry out a random check on the items in your shopping basket for 'hidden' helpings of artificial sweeteners: throat lozenges, vitamin pills and cough medicines are all common culprits – and they are all purportedly health-enhancing purchases.

right IT IS WISE ALWAYS TO USE HONEY SPARINGLY BECAUSE, HOWEVER NATURAL, IT IS STILL A FORM OF SUGAR.

Kicking the Caffeine Habit

In any concerted effort to reduce stress-related symptoms, we need to take an honest look at the amount of caffeine we are consuming regularly. Anyone who is drinking more than two cups of coffee and three cups of tea each day is definitely exceeding an advisable daily intake. If we also count the odd bar of plain chocolate and a couple of cans of caffeinated fizzy drinks, we can see that this is way out of line when it comes to managing caffeine levels.

In an ideal stress-free world, we could all cut out caffeine entirely, put up our feet and get through a day or two of caffeine-withdrawal symptoms and never have a cup of the delicious brew again. Life is stressful, however, and I, personally, enjoy an occasional cup of coffee. What we need to consider here, then, is a way of keeping our caffeine intake within reasonable limits. Aim to have no more than two cups of fresh coffee per day, and try to stick to one on most days.

If you feel the need for something hot as a matter of habit, there are plenty of low- or non-caffeinated alternatives available: matte tea, green tea, fruit-based mixtures, herbal teas (try to experiment with lemon verbena or the pleasantly aniseed-flavoured fennel, rather than predictably always opting for peppermint or camomile), or even grain-based coffee substitutes.

If, as I did in the past, you drink nine or ten mugs of strong coffee each day, you must be prepared for a 'cold turkey' withdrawal reaction. Classic caffeine withdrawal takes the form of a severe headache that can last as long as 24 hours, potentially compounded by feelings of slight queasiness and irritability. If you plan ahead and do this over a quiet weekend so that you can take it easy and wait for the reaction to pass, it will be more bearable. You must drink lots of water (still mineral or filtered) and fresh fruit juices. This will keep your system hydrated and help to flush away toxic waste in double-quick time.

If you prefer to adopt a less drastic plan of action, cut down your intake gradually and steadily

by two caffeinated cups a day, replacing them with any of the alternatives mentioned above. Once you are down to just one cup of fresh coffee a day, be ever watchful that the number does not start to creep back up. If this does keep happening, it may be that you are the type of person who has to junk caffeine altogether.

Fizzy cola drinks do nothing for us in health terms, and we would do well to give them up. There are lots of delicious alternatives available: try a fizzy mineral water with a dash of lemon or lime, or a carbonated spritzer with added fresh-fruit flavourings. Or try blending your own health-giving 'smoothies' or cocktails by juicing your favourite combinations of fresh fruit and vegetables.

Look closely at the labels of some so-called 'energy' drinks. Many of these contain caffeine and huge doses of sugar, and are best avoided if you want more sustained energy levels.

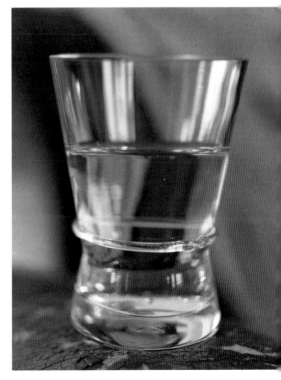

right GUARD AGAINST LOW-LEVEL DEHYDRATION BECOMING A PROBLEM BY DRINKING AT LEAST FOUR OR FIVE GLASSES OF WATER EVERY DAY.

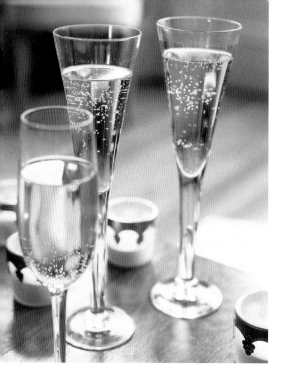

the days leading up to their period. Because of the depressant and mood-enhancing properties that alcohol is known to possess, they may suffer from rapid mood changes and a general sense of feeling emotionally low and depressed.

In order to get our alcohol consumption within realistic boundaries, we must be very honest when we assess how many units of alcohol we currently drink in an average week – with one unit being the equivalent of one measure of spirits, a small glass of wine or half a pint of beer. If women discover that they are exceeding their recommended maximum 14 units a week, and if men are beyond 21 units each week, it is time to take action.

Before we start, it is worth bearing in mind that there is a very good chance, if we are under a great deal of negative stress and pressure, that in addition to drinking too much (for its initially relaxing effect), we are probably also eating erratically and not very well, and possibly also smoking to help us unwind. If this scenario sounds uncannily familiar, it would be wise to invest in a good-quality multivitamin and multimineral supplement that will compensate for the vitamins and minerals that are depleted by smoking and drinking. If you have also suffered from recurrent colds since being stressed, it would help to take an extra 500 mg of vitamin C daily for a month.

In order to reap the maximum benefit from these supplements, you must take a break from alcohol altogether for a couple of weeks. This is important because it will give your overworked liver a much-needed rest and a chance to begin to recuperate.

There is no reason to feel severely restricted, because the days when an orange juice was pretty much the only non-alcoholic drink available have long gone. Sparkling, naturally fruit-flavoured and herbal non-alcoholic drinks provide an excellent alternative to wine with a meal, while most bars now also serve alcohol-free cocktails. These latter are a particularly clever ploy, because they look and taste much the

Kicking the Alcohol Habit

Although moderate quantities of alcohol can bring some health-protective benefits (a glass of red wine each day, it has been suggested, has a beneficial effect on the heart and circulatory system), if taken in excess it can have a seriously detrimental effect on our health. Violent mood swings, visible signs of premature ageing, diminished mental performance, disrupted sleep, liver damage and increased risk of thinning bones (osteoporosis): these are all problems known to be linked to high alcohol consumption.

As with caffeine, we need to develop a healthy way of managing our alcohol intake so that we stay within the recommended daily consumption. Women have a lower recommended weekly unit allowance than men: just 14 units as opposed to a man's 21. This is a consequence of the way in which men and women are known to metabolize alcohol differently – a fact due, in turn, to women having a different distribution and higher percentage of body fat.

Many women may also find that they are more sensitive and reactive to the effects of alcohol in same as the alcoholic variety, but allow us to avoid the drawbacks that come in the wake of alcohol. There is always sparkling mineral water, too, of course.

When you do return to drinking alcohol, make it a firm priority to stay well within the recommended unit allowance. Ideally, aim for three or four alcohol-free evenings every few weeks in order to give your liver an opportunity to recover and regenerate itself.

Kicking the Nicotine Habit

Smoking is acknowledged to be one of the toughest addictions to break, but any effort involved in giving up is well rewarded in terms of our health. Those of us who smoke significantly increase our chances of developing cancer of the lungs, heart and circulatory problems, bronchitis, osteoporosis, high blood pressure and signs of premature ageing. In addition, as we have seen, although initially it can make us feel relaxed, in the long term smoking appears to activate the stress response. Also, because of nicotine's highly addictive nature, if we go for too long without a cigarette, we will begin to feel irritable, jittery and on edge.

I have seen many succeed in giving up smoking during my experience as a homeopathic practitioner: some have used nicotine patches as a way of making the transition, while others have preferred an 'all-or-nothing' approach. If you are going through the process of trying to give up, it is worth remembering that alternative therapies, such as traditional Chinese medicine or Western medical herbalism, acupuncture, hypnotherapy and homeopathy, can be very helpful.

In any successful attempt to give up smoking, however, the single most important factor is the need to feel committed to your decision to give up. If you are trying to quit smoking primarily to please someone else, or are making only a half-hearted stab, success is likely to elude you. If, on the other hand, you are firmly resolved, and this determination is aided by any of the support mechanisms mentioned, the outcome is much more likely to be positive.

It can be very beneficial during an attempt to stop smoking to give your body additional support by taking some nutritional supplements. Not only do they help the body to recover, by disposing of toxic waste more efficiently, some of them can also support the nervous system, which will help to combat the feelings of agitation or irritability that generally accompany withdrawal.

Kicking the Painkiller Habit

Anyone suffering from recurrent headaches should check what sort of painkiller they tend to use: the powerful paracetamol and codeine combinations that are available over the counter could, in fact, be contributing to the problem. These painkillers, because of the highly addictive nature of the codeine component, may cause 'rebound' headaches.

Try exploring effective but less aggressive ways of treating headaches (see pages 109–111), but if you do need to resort to a painkiller, try a paracetamol-only formula, staying strictly within the recommended dose.

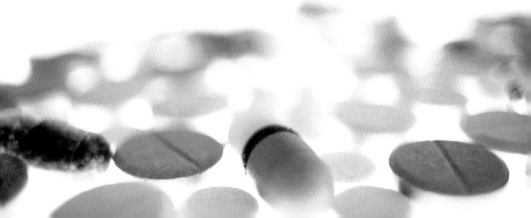

Blood-Sugar Levels and Burnout

It has already been established that blood-sugar levels play an extremely important role in helping us maintain a sense of mental, emotional and physical balance. If we suffer from constantly fluctuating blood-sugar levels that plunge rapidly from unadvisably high to unreasonably low, we are sure to suffer from a host of unpleasant symptoms. Unfortunately, however, realizing – or working out – where the root of the problem lies can take some time and effort.

This is especially true if we are also coping with large amounts of negative stress, as symptoms commonly associated with low blood-sugar levels (hypoglycaemia) can closely mimic stress-related problems – any, or any combination, of the following:

- Headaches
- Drowsiness
- Irritability
- A sense of panic under pressure
- Palpitations
- Food cravings
- General aches and pains
- A reduced ability to concentrate

Balancing Blood Sugar

Most of us might think that if these problems are initiated or made worse by having blood-sugar levels that are too low, the obvious solution would be to make sure that we get a good regular dose of sugar. Unfortunately, this is probably, in fact, the worst thing we could do.

When we feed ourselves generous amounts of sugar on a regular basis our bodies respond by secreting enough insulin to reduce our blood-sugar levels. It is the job of the pancreas to 'police' our blood-sugar levels and to decide when, and how much, insulin is required to keep these levels within desirable boundaries. Unfortunately, if we throw excessive sugar at our pancreas too often, the poor organ eventually becomes trigger-happy and

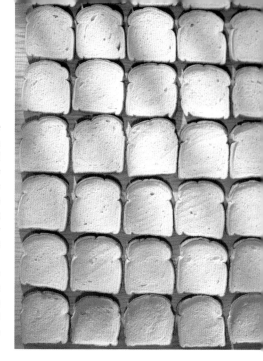

exhausted. If this routine is left unchecked for too long, it can result in maturity-onset diabetes (often referred to as 'type-two' diabetes).

Maturity-onset diabetes is usually diagnosed in middle age, and is probably the consequence of eating too many foods made from refined carbohydrates for too many years: things like white bread, white rice, white pasta, cakes, cookies and snack-type products (both sweet and savoury). These are problem items from the blood-sugar-level perspective because they contain high amounts of white sugar and flour, as well as – often – a hefty proportion of fat. The situation can be made much worse if liberal doses of white sugar are added, in the form of hot drinks, fizzy sodas and colas, plenty of sweets, chocolate and sticky puddings.

Before we reach this stage, however, fluctuating blood-sugar levels can cause all sorts of problems: mental and emotional fatigue; energy levels that go up and down with alarming rapidity; and regular or constant cravings for sweet and salty things. The latter is a sure sign that the pancreas is being overenthusiastic: as blood-sugar levels are brought down too dramatically, we are left feeling exhausted and craving another sugar 'fix'. It is a vicious circle

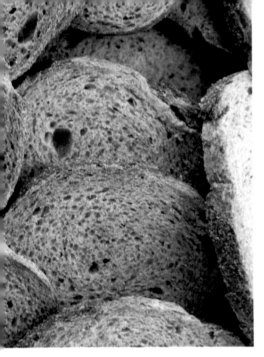

left FIBRE-RICH WHOLEMEAL BREAD SHOULD ALWAYS BE CHOSEN IN PREFERENCE TO REFINED WHITE BREAD.

Ultimately, you can safely choose to include any of the following in a diet designed to keep blood-sugar levels steady:

- Wholegrain products of any kind, which includes bread, oats, pasta and rice. Complex, unrefined carbohydrates of this sort are broken down more slowly than their refined relatives, so they help to create more stable, less erratic energy levels
- Fresh fruit, ideally in its basic state and not juiced; juicing removes the fibre from fruit yet the fibrous content effectively works as a 'buffer', preventing the fruit sugar from raising blood-sugar levels too precipitately
- Small amounts of protein: poultry, milk, cheese, yogurt (either natural or with fresh fruit added) and soya
- Nuts and seeds
- Fresh vegetables of all kinds and varieties
- Pulses: beans and lentils
- Oily fish, such as mackerel, sardines and salmon, contain important fatty acids that help to protect our hearts and circulatory systems

that will inevitably end in pancreatic exhaustion if left unmanaged. The good news, however, is that this undesirable scenario can be averted if action is taken early enough.

The trick is to be aware of the problem, and to make sure that foods and drinks that balance our blood-sugar levels become a staple part of our daily diet.

Blood-Sugar Stabilizers

Before we consider the types of food and drink that can help to keep blood-sugar levels as steady as possible, it is also important to bear in mind that the frequency and regularity with which we eat also has a beneficial or detrimental effect on blood-sugar stability. The ideal eating pattern for guarding against plummeting blood-sugar levels involves making sure that we eat 'a little something' every couple of hours.

'Little' really does mean little in this context. It need be no more than a piece of fruit or a slice of wholemeal bread or a wholewheat cracker. Anything made from refined, white sugar, on the other hand, whether it comes in the form of a cube of chocolate or a fizzy drink, should be avoided.

Treat the following with caution:

- Anything made from white flour and sugar, including white bread, sweets, chocolate, cakes, cookies and puddings
- Alcohol
- Sweetened fizzy drinks
- Fruit squashes – flavoured syrups that are diluted with water
- Junk food that bears no resemblance at all to its natural state, such as chicken nuggets
- Anything that contains large amounts of 'hidden' sugar: canned tomato soup, baked beans and ketchup are common culprits
- Chocolate
- Coffee: when drunk frequently, even with no sugar added to it, coffee plays havoc with blood-sugar levels. As a result, once its initial stimulating effect has worn off, it can – like sugar – contribute to mood swings, fatigue and poor concentration

Convenience Foods

It is generally accepted that too heavy a reliance on convenience foods is likely to give rise to a number of recognized problems. The reality of running a busy professional and home life simultaneously, however, means that there are inevitably times when a catering crisis requires a stop-gap solution. Convenience foods provide us with precisely that sort of buffer when time is tight: an entire meal ready in half an hour at the end of the day.

What we need to do, ideally, is discover ways to minimize any damage caused by eating ready-made meals, while ensuring that we vary the nature of what we eat as frequently as possible.

The best policy is to call basic common sense into play: if a food is brightly and unnaturally coloured, heavily processed or rendered unrecognizable from its natural state, it is generally advisable to resist temptation and avoid it.

below **TOMATO KETCHUP CAN CONTAIN A SIGNIFICANT AMOUNT OF 'HIDDEN' SUGAR.**

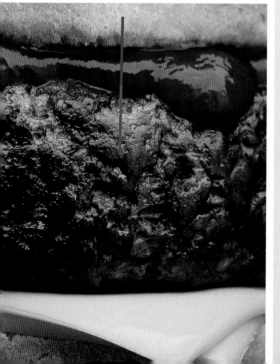

Troubleshooting Hints

- Avoid eating anything that no longer resembles its original source and anything that has been thoroughly processed. Just one look at the sell by/eat by dates of vacuum-packed items will give a clear indication of how woefully lacking in freshness the ingredients will be.
- Foods that have had their shelf life disturbingly extended by chemical preservatives, and their appearance and taste 'assisted' by chemical colourings and flavourings, should also be studiously avoided – chemicals used as preservatives can adversely affect bone density.
- Avoid anything that has been heavily salted, smoked or charred. All these processes can contribute to problems with high blood pressure, while smoked or charred foods may also have potentially carcinogenic properties when eaten regularly or in large quantities.
- Focus on foods that have not been messed about with: portions of fresh chicken or fish that simply need to be grilled or marinated, for example.
- Make sure you eat at least five portions of fresh fruit and vegetables every day. Fitting them in is easy if you have one piece of fruit at breakfast, a generous salad at lunchtime with fresh fruit afterwards; a piece of fruit mid-afternoon, and two or three vegetables at dinner followed by another generous portion of fruit.
- Avoid microwaving convenience foods in their plastic containers when you are heating them. While it may take a little longer to transfer the food into a glass container, the benefits are well worth the effort. It has been suggested that oestrogen-type chemicals can leach from the plastic container into the food in the heat of the microwave. Xenoestrogens, as these chemicals are called, have been implicated in a whole host of health problems, including muzzy-headedness, premenstrual tension, hormone imbalances and a general sense of fatigue.

Extra Support: Essential Nutritional Supplements

We should generally be aiming to obtain the full spectrum of essential nutrients daily simply by eating sensibly, according to the guidelines given previously. However, there will inevitably be times when life seems to go off the rails, and during these phases a booster course of supplements can give us the impetus we need to get ourselves back on track. Indeed, a number of key nutrients have been found to play a very important role in helping to safeguard us against the pernicious effects of protracted negative stress.

VITAMIN C

Indisputably a 'wonder' vitamin, vitamin C helps the body to fight off infection efficiently; protects against free-radical damage (free radicals are rampaging molecules that contribute to the development of an extensive range of degenerative conditions, including heart disease and hardening of the arteries); maintains the health and good condition of the skin; and generally shortens the duration of any infectious illnesses. It is clearly itself a nutrient that we need to take in every day.

It is fairly easy in summer to eat plenty of foods rich in vitamin C. After all, tucking in to large amounts of salad, fresh fruit, fresh juices and plenty of vegetables is hardly a hardship in hot weather. The winter months, however, might prove more difficult, because many of us instinctively gravitate towards a more substantial diet at this time of the year. It is also important to remember that vitamin C is very volatile. It is water-soluble, which means that supplies cannot be built up and stored in the body. It is, therefore, absolutely vital that we take in enough vitamin C every day.

If we cut open an orange and leave it for two hours before we eat or juice it, its vitamin-C content will have dropped dramatically in the interim. Because it oxidizes readily when it comes into contact with the atmosphere, vitamin C is easily destroyed. The same is true of salad vegetables, such as raw peppers or tomatoes. Valuably rich in vitamin C, these should be prepared at the very last minute in order to avoid precious vitamin C leaching away. Cooking methods should also be as quick and light as possible for similar reasons: steaming is the best of all.

If we have been turning to alcohol and excessive numbers of cigarettes in an attempt to deal with ever mounting negative stress levels, we need to look to vitamin C for help. Alcohol and cigarettes impair the effective absorption of vitamin C at the very time when we are likely to need this vitamin most. Suffering from a series of minor infections following one another in quick succession, often after a period when we have been burning the candle at both ends, is clear evidence that our body is crying out for vitamin C.

If this unhappy scenario sounds familiar to you, it is evidently time to increase the amount of vitamin C-rich foods and drinks in your daily diet. It should

above **AVOID CHOPPING VITAMIN C-RICH FRUIT OR VEGETABLES HOURS BEFORE THEY ARE DUE TO BE EATEN, AS VITAMIN C OXIDIZES AND BREAKS DOWN ON CONTACT WITH AIR.**

not be too hard, as any of the following would be considered beneficial:

- Berries, such as blackcurrants and blueberries
- Strawberries
- Citrus fruit, including oranges, grapefruit, lemons and satsumas
- Kiwi fruit
- Dark green vegetables, including broccoli and Brussels sprouts
- Cauliflower
- Tomatoes
- Raw peppers, red and green

If you have been under stress for an extended period, taking vitamin C in supplement form will also be helpful. Take 1 g (1,000 mg) each day for the first two weeks; unless you are taking a slow-release formula, it is best to take four 250 mg doses spread throughout the day. This is a practical measure designed to optimize the benefits of the dose, because the vitamin lingers in the body for only a relatively short time. A series of easily assimilable small hits is better than 1g in a single dose as you start the day, because later in the day most of that will already have been flushed out of your body.

After two weeks you can probably cut down to a maintenance dose of 500 mg per day, which – generally – you can continue until you feel you are back on an even keel. If, however, any signs of bowel intolerance occur (an acid stomach and/or diarrhoea), you should further reduce the dose.

VITAMIN B COMPLEX

The B vitamins, including thiamin, riboflavin, niacin, folate and B12, have been shown to play an essential role in supporting the nervous system, and the need for this support becomes particularly acute at times of stress and strain. The B vitamins boost neural activation, and vitamin B12 specifically has been shown to facilitate the normal metabolism of chemicals that help to prevent depression. Vitamin B6 has attracted a great deal of publicity lately, too, as an enormously beneficial supplement for women who suffer from the debilitating symptoms of premenstrual syndrome.

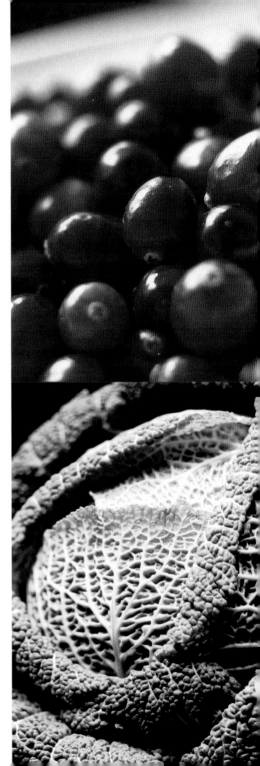

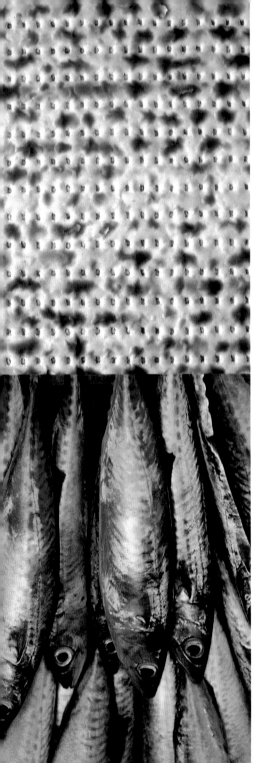

left VARY YOUR INTAKE OF DIETARY INGREDIENTS AS MUCH AS POSSIBLE IN ORDER TO GUARD AGAINST GETTING BORED WITH FOOD – AND FOOD PREPARATION.

Although, like vitamin C, the B-complex vitamins are water-soluble and cannot be stored by the body, what has become clear is that an excessively high or unbalanced dose of one of the B-complex vitamins in isolation can give rise to fresh problems. The way to avoid this is to make sure that when you take a vitamin B supplement, it is made up of the whole complex, as each component appears to work best in conjunction with the others. Always buy a reputable brand that provides the full spectrum of B complex in a balanced formula, rather than cheaper versions that do not contain all the elements. Follow the suggested dosage for as long as stress levels continue to be high.

Make a point, too, when you know negative stress levels are high, of eating foods rich in vitamin B regularly. These include:

- Poultry
- Fish
- Nuts
- Seeds
- Wholegrain products, including wholewheat bread and pasta
- Red meat (sparingly)
- Soya products
- Potatoes
- Green, leafy vegetables
- Yeast extract

CALCIUM

When we are under stress our need for calcium increases. This is because the stress hormone noradrenaline is switched on as part of the stress response and when this happens regularly it encourages the excretion of calcium stores from our bones. If this continues to occur over an extended period, it will militate against our chances of maintaining healthy, strong bones. During and after the menopause women will feel especially vulnerable because thinning of the bones (osteoporosis) is a relatively common problem that often strikes at this stage in life as a result of hormonal changes.

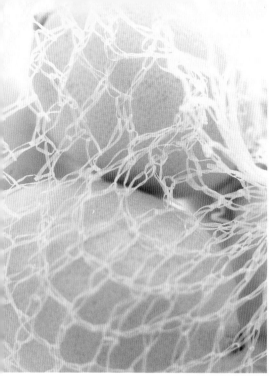

If you are considering taking a calcium supplement, it helps to remember that in order to maximize the chances of effective absorption you will also need to take magnesium and vitamin D. Bear in mind, too, that although calcium carbonate is the most common – and cheapest – variety of calcium available in supplement form, this does have the potential to introduce other problems: poor absorption, digestive upsets, breast nodules and an increased chance of kidney stones. For these reasons it is far better to choose a calcium citrate formula; it will be more readily absorbed by the body, and less likely to trigger unwanted side effects. And, for the same reasons, it is best to aim for a combined magnesium and calcium formula – ideally comprising twice as much magnesium as calcium.

If we want to boost our magnesium intake through wise food choices, the following will be helpful:

- Apples
- Nuts
- Seeds, particularly sesame seeds
- Figs
- Lemons
- Green vegetables

KAVA KAVA

Kava kava is attracting much attention as a non-addictive, herbal supplement that can help reduce stress-related symptoms – feelings of anxiety and of being mentally, emotionally and physically 'on edge'. Derived from the pepper family, kava kava has been used in the Pacific islands for many years as a soothing and relaxing drink. Unlike alcohol, it does not produce aggressive behaviour. Moreover, it appears to be tremendously effective in promoting a sound and refreshing night's sleep, without leaving the drowsy, 'hungover' feeling that is often associated with conventional sleeping pills.

Contained in kava kava are compounds called kavalactones. Studies have revealed that these active ingredients have an impressively wide range of sedative, pain-relieving and muscle-relaxing properties.

Menopause is known to be a stressful period, so it is clearly a priority for women approaching their late forties and early fifties – and particularly those who are under stress already – to explore ways of protecting their bone density. As well as finding ways to manage stress effectively, evaluating their calcium intake must be a primary consideration in this.

Calcium has also been shown to support the body as it deals with stress on other levels. It helps us to achieve a sound night's sleep; promotes balanced levels of potassium and sodium; lowers cholesterol levels in the blood; and helps to stabilize blood pressure. It also helps to prevent muscle cramps, especially if taken in combination with magnesium. Good dietary sources of calcium include:

- Dairy products, such as cheese and milk
- Canned fish, eaten with the bones intact
- Pulses
- Green, leafy vegetables
- Soya beans
- Sesame seeds
- Tofu

Although kavalactones seem to produce as powerful a calming effect as conventional tranquillizers, they function in a subtly and significantly different way.

Most conventional sedatives achieve their desired effect by affecting specific receptors in the brain. Kavalactones, on the other hand, seem to work on the limbic system. So far, studies have suggested that kavalactones can promote sound sleep by modifying the way in which our limbic systems control our emotions. It seems to be because they function in this different sphere of action that the sedative and pain-relieving effects of kava kava do not give rise to the dependency problems that appear inevitably to arise with conventional painkillers and tranquillizers. Its muscle-relaxant function makes kava kava especially helpful in easing tension headaches that arise from tightness in the neck and shoulders.

When taken in an appropriate dose, kava kava appears not to have any major side effects. Very high doses, however, can cause a thickening of the skin on the hands and the soles of the feet. And problems occur if this herbal supplement is taken with conventional antidepressants or tranquillizers. Never take both kinds at the same time, as the interaction between conventional sedatives and antidepressants and kava kava is potentially dangerous. If you are in any doubt about the safety of taking kava kava, always seek the opinion of your GP or pharmacist.

GINSENG

Ginseng appears to have important stress-proofing properties that can benefit our minds and bodies when they are exposed to an excessive amount of negative stress. In controlled studies ginseng has been shown to help to maintain the balance of neurotransmitters when we are under pressure. Not only does it effectively bar any increased production of brain cortisol (and increased cortisol can impair concentration), it also acts to bolster the feelgood chemicals serotonin and norepinephrine to prevent their levels dropping. This helps guard against the onslaught of feelings of depression

and negativity. Ginseng has also been shown to reduce levels of anxiety in response to stress.

Because ginseng has also been observed to play a significantly positive role in supporting our immune systems, this is an especially important supplement for us to consider if we feel physically run down when we are stressed. However, it is worth bearing in mind that, paradoxically, while moderate doses appear to give our immune systems a major boost, larger doses seem to have the reverse effect and actually inhibit the performance of the immune system.

Make a point of choosing the best-quality ginseng available, rather than going for a budget brand, if you want to reap the maximum benefits from this supplement. Inferior, cheaper products may yield very little of the active ingredient.

It is best to avoid taking ginseng on a routine, daily basis; instead, aim to take a two-week course, then leave a two-week gap before beginning another course. The optimum suggested daily dose is 200 mg – divided into two doses of 100 mg. If you are contemplating a course of ginseng, but have a history of high blood pressure, or cancer of the womb or breast, you should seek medical advice first.

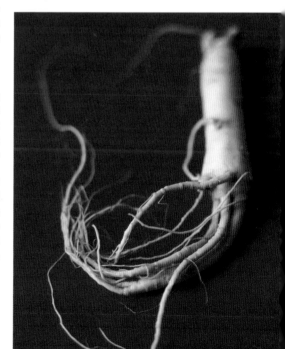

right **STRESS-RELATED SYMPTOMS MAY BENEFIT FROM SUPPLEMENTING THE DIET WITH GINSENG.**

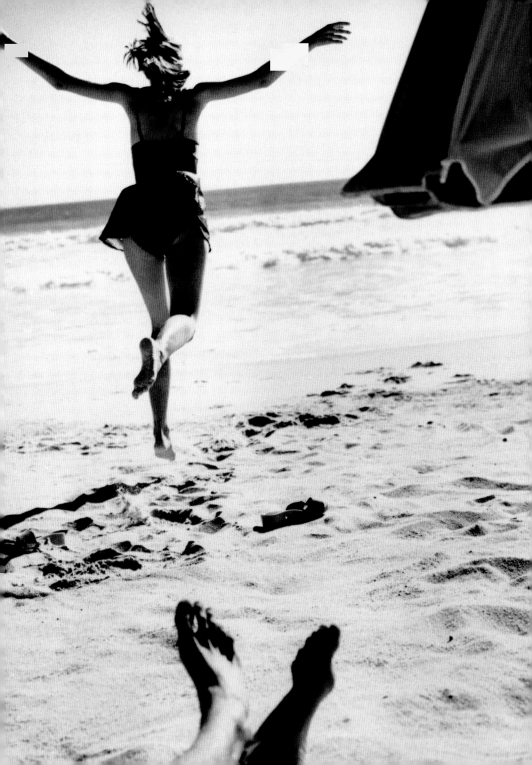

5 Replenish: Exercise to De-stress and Regain Optimum Health

Having spent my youth as a confirmed couch potato, it seems ironic 40 or so years later to be writing an enthusiastic chapter on the multiple benefits of physical fitness. However, this most unlikely transformation in my own attitude to fitness has a great deal to do with the way that exercise systems have been subject to rapidly changing trends over the past two decades.

Eventually – and thankfully – we have recently seen a new model of exercise emerge that is in sympathy with the current search for optimum emotional, mental and physical balance and harmony. This provides a fascinating contrast to the 'going for the burn' and 'no pain, no gain' mantras that were common currency in the 1980s. During that decade fitness and slimness were held up as the ultimate goals, while the reduction of stress and the general promotion of health – though obviously desirable – were essentially considered optional extra bonuses. Surface appearances were paramount, and even if an exercise regime was harsh, povided that the cosmetic advantages were substantial it tended to become flavour of the month.

Mercifully, there has been welcome progress in the fitness world, and if we want to get ourselves in better physical shape today we can choose from

a range of exercise systems that are as much concerned with restoring our emotional and mental wellbeing and resilience as they are able to tone, lengthen and strengthen unfit muscles.

The chapter is called Replenish because all the physical activities it discusses have been chosen deliberately for their stress-reducing, mood-balancing and energy-regulating potential. Rather than draining our energy reserves, these systems of movement all come with established reputations for building mental, emotional and physical resilience, making it easier for us to cope with any of life's punches.

The Benefits of Regular Exercise

Enjoyable, regular exercise is a strong ally in any struggle for effective stress-busting – for two very different reasons. Firstly, vigorous, rhythmic physical movement gives our bodies a chance to 'burn off' excess adrenaline and any additional stress hormones that might be circulating in our systems as part of the fight-or-flight response. Secondly, exercise will help to reduce the tension and stiffness that builds up in our muscles, particularly in the muscles of the face, neck and shoulders if our lifestyle is overloaded with

left REGULAR, ENJOYABLE EXERCISE CAN HELP TO STIMULATE IMPROVED LEVELS OF ENERGY AND VITALITY.

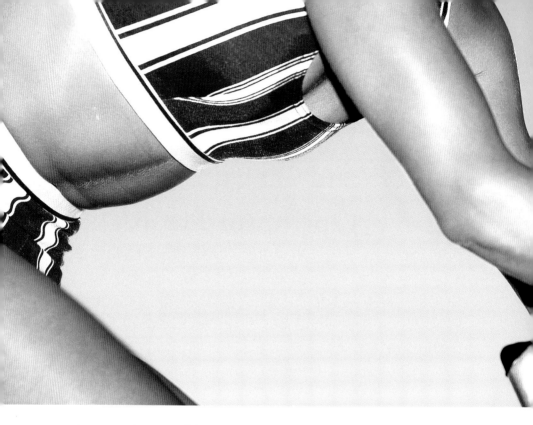

negative stress and pressure. If this tension were allowed to become established, the stage would be set for the frequent and regular appearance of stress-related tension headaches and other such debilitating chronic complaints.

The regular practice of mind/body balancing systems such as yoga, T'ai chi or Qi gong has an added bonus in the stress-reduction stakes, because any of these will teach us gentle ways to switch off and relax – particularly helpful if we have a tendency to get irritable and tense at a moment's notice, or if we are having problems being able to relax sufficiently at night to enjoy sound, restful sleep.

Not only helping us to process the stress chemicals that flood our systems when we are under pressure, physical exercise also brings positive benefits to our circulatory system, effecting the efficient transportation of oxygen and nutrients to each cell in our bodies. Importantly, too, however, regular physical activity can have either a tranquillizing

or an energizing effect; we can choose which form of exercise to take at any given time, depending on the desired effect.

Regular exercise thus has an impressive range of benefits that help to condition our bodies and also support us in our campaign to deal more effectively with negative stress.

Fringe Benefits: Lifting the Spirits

Over the past decade it has become apparent that the more holistic model of exercise has an extra dimension. This aspect relates to the positive effects of exercise on the mind and emotions.

If we exercise regularly, there is a good chance that we will experience a huge increase in self-esteem and self-confidence – a direct consequence of actually taking control and taking action. In contrast, it is very demoralizing to be aware that our bodies are crying out for attention, but to lack the motivation or resolve to do anything about it. Summoning that motivation is amply repaid: knowing that we possess a strong, flexible body that moves easily, free from pain, tension or stiffness, brings a priceless sense of sheer pleasure.

Beyond these feelgood factors, however, there is one basic, physiological change that occurs in our bodies when we exercise regularly, one that plays a significant part in stimulating a profound sense of wellbeing. When we exercise rhythmically and aerobically for a sustained period, naturally occurring, feelgood chemicals are secreted into the bloodstream. They are called endorphins. It is widely believed that these endorphins are responsible for the sense of elation that is known to follow a stint of aerobic walking, swimming or cycling. Endorphins are believed to be naturally occurring antidepressants with a calming, sedative effect.

It is now recognized that regular aerobic exercise can play a significant and important part in helping us deal with mild or moderate feelings of anxiety and depression. Indeed, one exercise laboratory in California has suggested that a regular, brisk walk can have as significant a calming effect as 400 mg of a chemical tranquilliser.

There are generally recognized problems that may arise if tranquillizers or antidepressants are relied upon to control anxiety and minor depression – potential side effects, too. So it is easy to see how advantageous it is to consider taking up regular exercise as a first resort (in an attempt to improve our mental and emotional balance), rather than feeling obliged automatically to go down the conventional medication route. It will give us an important sense of having taken some control, which in turn will help to dispel, a little, some of the feelings of lack of confidence and helplessness that generally accompany feeling tense or 'blue'.

left and right **WHETHER ACTIVE CYCLING OR RELAXING YOGA APPEALS, CHOOSE AN EXERCISE REGIME THAT SUITS YOU AND YOUR LIFESTYLE.**

Creative Possibilities: Combination Exercises

Rather than an exhaustive survey of the most up-to-date exercise regimes available, what follows is a basic guide to some of the most established and effective systems of movement that have earned a 'tried-and-tested' reputation for increasing strength and stamina while also imparting a sense of mental and emotional wellbeing.

Yoga

Experiencing today a huge resurgence in general interest, yoga is one of the oldest and best-known movement systems for promoting harmony of body and mind. Although we tend to speak about yoga as a single entity, there are in fact several different forms; which one we choose to pursue will depend on our level of fitness, and on what we hope to gain.

If, basically, we want to tone up our muscles, build up our strength, increase our flexibility, and learn how to use our breathing to relax or revitalize, Hatha yoga will probably be the most suitable type, especially for the beginner.

Iyengar yoga is both much more demanding in the physical sense and requires great precision and accuracy if maximum benefit is to be gained from each posture.

Anyone who is already physically fit and who wants a fast-moving class with a reputation for fat-burning should explore 'Power' or Astanga Vinyasa yoga, which may prove a more suitable choice than those branches of the system described above. Regular practice of Astanga Vinyasa yoga will provide not only a good level of cardiovascular fitness but a sleek, slim, strong and incredibly flexible body, too.

Yoga is a system of exercise that can teach us how to use our breathing for effective stress release, while also calming feelings of tension and anxiety. All forms of yoga involve learning to develop a keen awareness of breath control in order to gain the maximum benefit from each posture. In addition, practised regularly, yoga will increase energy levels, promote tranquillity of the mind, increase stamina, enhance flexibility and muscle tone and strength, and improve circulation. Healing energy will be able to flow freely to all parts of the body. If we make yoga a regular part of our lives, we will be giving ourselves one of the most comprehensive, top-to-toe workouts available.

To learn how to do yoga correctly, it is essential to attend a regular class – it is the only way to master the basic postures. It is fine to practise at home once you become more adept, and there is an increasing range of helpful videos available. For basic advice on all aspects of yoga, and to find a class, contact a yoga organization (see Address Book, page 124).

It is wise to remember that our needs can change over the years. We may, for example, have tried yoga when we were younger and we may have decided that it was not an appropriate system of exercise for us, but it is still worth giving it another chance now. Alternatively, we may – when we were unaware of the different branches of yoga – have been advised to try Hatha yoga and not realized that once we had mastered this, we could advance to the more fast-moving approach found in Astanga yoga if we wanted the challenge provided by this demanding form.

right THE FOCUS OF A YOGA SESSION WILL LEAVE YOU FEELING REVITALIZED AND INTEGRATED — YOUR MIND AND BODY WILL BE WORKING IN HARMONY.

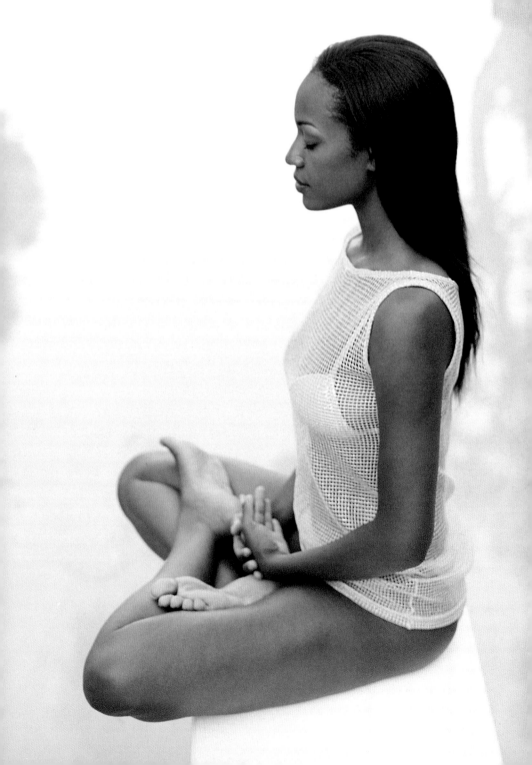

Pilates

Originally developed by Joseph Pilates in the 1920s as a physiotherapeutic system of movement, Pilates classes have become immensely popular in the past ten years. Those who want to find a system of exercise that helps reduce the negative effects of physical, emotional and mental stress, while also providing a fitness programme that promotes a longer, leaner shape should consider exploring the Pilates technique. This form of exercise requires multiple repetitions of controlled, precise movements that isolate and work specific muscle groups.

When Pilates is taught well and practised regularly, the benefits can be wide-ranging and impressive: improved posture, leaner muscles, enhanced muscle tone, increased flexibility, and greater mental and emotional balance. Because a considerable level of concentration needs to be brought to play to execute these exercises correctly, and because there is throughout a focus on breathing steadily and deeply – lowering the heart rate and blood pressure – regular practise of Pilates can also play an important role in any stress-reduction programme.

Pilates classes concentrate on building a point of core stability, focusing on the area extending from the bottom of the rib cage to the area between the hip bones. Some exercises are executed standing upright, others lying on a mat, and some classes will use special Pilates equipment.

It is very important for beginners to attend a class in order to understand fully what they are attempting to do, because Pilates exercises require precision and accuracy to be effective. Once you have learnt the intention behind each exercise, practising at home will accelerate your progress and build on the headway made in class.

Qi gong

Qi gong has been mooted as one of the most relaxing and beneficial systems of movement we can perform to help alleviate stress-related problems. It is hailed as being especially beneficial for those who feel that they need to learn how to focus mentally and then how to maintain their concentration once they have attained it.

Qi gong teaches you how to breathe regularly and deeply while performing

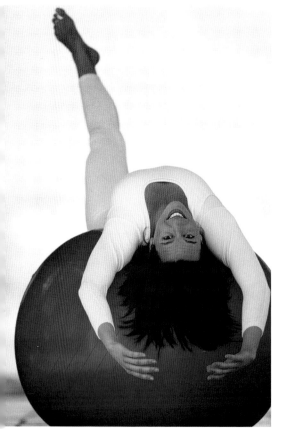

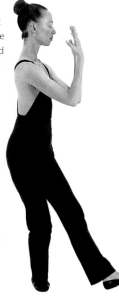

left PILATES CONCENTRATES ON BUILDING A SENSE OF BODY AWARENESS. right WHEN PRACTISED REGULARLY, QI GONG CAN HELP TO INDUCE A PROFOUND SENSE OF MENTAL FOCUS.

a series of gentle, flowing exercises involving slow, repetitive movements. As you are doing these exercises you are encouraged to focus the mind. This ensures that you will not be distracted by stressful thoughts during Qi gong practice.

As you become more adept at this stress-reducing technique, you should find that you experience bigger energy reserves, improved overall health (as a result of more efficient immune-system performance), and improved muscular coordination and strength.

Although introductory books and videos on Qi gong are available, it is advisable initially to seek out private tuition from a traditional Chinese practitioner or to attend a Qi gong class. This will guarantee that you are executing the movements correctly and deriving maximum benefit from them.

The Alexander Technique

Although this is not strictly an exercise system, a quick explanation of the Alexander Technique is especially relevant to any discussion of stress reduction and stress management. This is because practitioners of the Alexander Technique concentrate on teaching their pupils how to break the negative postural habits that they have been unconsciously developing over a number of years. Learning how to identify and break these postural habits can be especially liberating to people who respond to stressful situations by unconsciously tensing up their muscles and distorting their posture. It is these negative postural habits that, in the long term, can lead to recurrent tension headaches, back pain and generalized stiffness, tension and inflexibility in the joints and muscles.

From the perspective of the Alexander Technique, not only does the way we feel have a profound effect on our posture, but conversely, too, the way we hold ourselves has a strong effect on our emotions and frame of mind. For instance, if we feel tense and anxious, we are likely to find that we clench our jaw, and our neck and shoulder muscles may tighten and become rigid. On the other hand, if our eyes are constantly drawn towards the floor and we instinctively adopt a sagging posture, with our shoulders hunched forwards, we are likely to find that we lack confidence and feel low or depressed a great deal of the time. Moreover, because maintaining these postural habits actually uses up a great deal of energy, they can contribute to generally lacklustre feelings of lethargy and weariness. This is only the negative side of the situation, however.

As soon as we realize that we should change this pattern, we can begin upon a liberating journey of discovery and self-awareness, on which we can deal much more effectively with anxious or tense situations by consciously changing our posture. We will also find that feelings of anxiety or depression diminish as we become more aware of our bodies and learn how to carry ourselves in an altogether more balanced, relaxed way. In other words, if we can influence our posture by how we feel, we can also affect how we feel by altering our postural habits.

It is important to be prepared for well-established, ingrained postural habits to be more difficult to break than we might initially expect. It is quite likely that we will catch ourselves longing to return to the way in which we held ourselves before – even though it was probably having a negative effect – simply because it feels more comfortable to us than the newer, more positive postural habits. It is definitely worth persevering, however, because once we are familiar with how to practise the Alexander Technique, we will be armed with an effective and practical tool that we can use to advantage in times of extreme pressure and emotional crisis.

The Alexander Technique needs to be learnt from a trained practitioner; it is not worth trying to master the method by yourself from a book. Classes are usually given on a personal-tuition basis, with the tutor spending a major proportion of the lesson time observing the way in which you carry yourself as you execute simple, everyday movements – sitting down, or getting out of a chair, for example. Once tuition is underway, a teacher will usually suggest additional exercises that can be done regularly at home.

T'ai chi

T'ai chi developed in China as a martial art more than 1,000 years ago. Since then it has gained a reputation as a system of meditation in movement that has the potential to balance energy levels and stimulate greater harmony between mind, emotions and body. Regular practice of T'ai chi should promote an enhanced sense of tranquillity, greater confidence and improved muscle tone.

T'ai chi comprises the execution of a series of continuous flowing movements while breathing consciously and regularly. It is thought that the practice of T'ai chi stimulates an improved flow of energy through the body, while at the same time relaxing the muscles and improving circulation. Increased joint mobility; better toned, more flexible muscles; and improved posture are sometimes also claimed as additional benefits of T'ai chi. All in all, in common with Qi gong, T'ai chi should engender improvements in general physical balance and coordination if performed regularly.

As with other systems, it is very important to attend a T'ai chi class to learn how to perform the basic movements correctly; practising a system inaccurately will seriously undermine the potential benefits to be gained from it.

Because T'ai chi encourages an awareness of breathing patterns, it can be especially helpful to those of us who hyperventilate when feeling stressed or anxious. Being aware of how we breathe is the crucial first step towards being able to alter such negative patterns in times of stress in the future.

below **T'AI CHI CAN HELP IMPROVE GENERAL BALANCE AND MUSCULAR COORDINATION.** right **TRY TO MAKE REGULAR EXERCISE AN INTEGRAL PART OF YOUR DAY.**

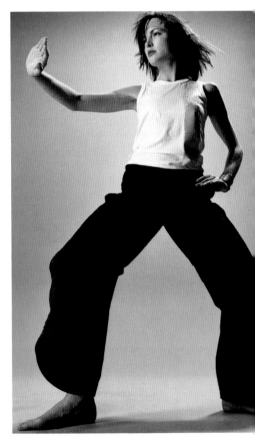

Making it Work: Integrating Exercise into our Lives

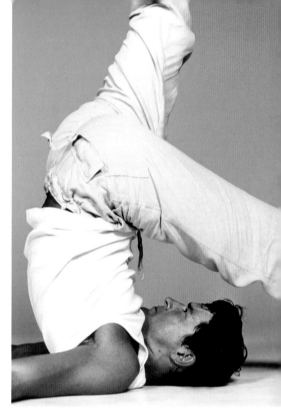

- The first rule of successfully integrating any fitness regime into our lives is to keep things as simple as possible. Many people feel that they have to take radical action in order to get themselves fit. It is precisely this sort of mind-set that persuades us to take out a subscription to a smart gym after Christmas, full of good intentions to go along four nights a week to get back into great physical shape in time for summer. Unfortunately, this is the type of approach that often leads to failure, because we are overambitious about the commitment that we intend to make: a flurry of activity in the gym for a few weeks dwindles to nothing as other regular calls on our time begin to reassert themselves. What is worse, however, is that this sort of well-intentioned but basically unrealistic programme leaves us with a lurking sense of guilt, which serves only to increase levels of negative stress rather than diminishing them.

- Always make sure you know the best time of day for you to exercise. We all have different body clocks and constitutions and, as a result, some of us will be at our best early in the morning before we start the routines of our day, while others will find the early evening far more appropriate. Developing this sense of awareness is useful in itself: learning what suits our bodies will make us more in tune with ourselves generally.

- Be truly realistic about the amount of time you can devote to your exercise regime, and take into account in your calculations that you are making a long-term commitment, not indulging in a passing phase. If you are realistic and not overambitious, you should find that you will be able to keep your fitness programme going. Always bear in mind that establishing a regular routine is probably the best – and easiest – way of sticking successfully to a fitness programme. Once you have established a regular routine, you are very likely to find that you actually want to devote more time to your fitness regime, because you will have begun to see and feel the many benefits that result from regular exercise. Letting an exercise programme develop slowly and steadily in an organic way will prove worthwhile; as it changes and grows, your interest will be sustained and, in consequence, the chances are that you will want to maintain the impetus and will keep at it.

- Most important of all, give thought to choosing a system of exercise, or a combination, that complements your temperament, taste and interests. There is, after all, little point in forcing yourself to attend a T'ai chi class if you would really rather be swimming. Conversely, however, do give new systems of movement a chance and see how you respond to them. If you begin to feel bored or uninspired, alter your course and try something different; otherwise there is a very strong danger that you will be so demoralized as to give up exercise altogether.

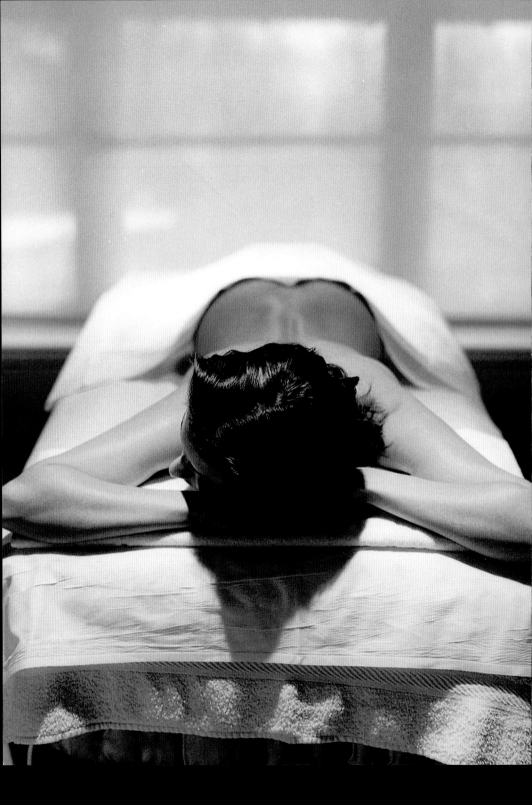

6

Pamper:
Melt Away Stress
with Body Treats

We all need a thorough pampering from time to time, and this chapter reveals the de-stressing benefits of luxuriating in some basic body treats. Before such indulgence begins to sound a little too hedonistic and guilt-inducing, it is very important to bear in mind that pleasurable experiences (apart from being delightful for their own sake) have been observed to have a beneficial effect on our health.

Stressful experiences have been shown to have a markedly negative effect, leaving us more vulnerable to illnesses such as high blood pressure, irritable bowel syndrome and degenerative heart disease. Pleasurable experiences, on the other hand, appear to carry important health benefits. Experiments have shown that while our immune systems can be depressed by the recollection of stressful or distressing memories, deliberately recalling pleasurable memories can actually boost the immune system. In the same way, laughter, making love and exposure to pleasing sensual impressions seem generally to benefit our health.

As stress-related problems tend to become more intense when we have too little time for ourselves, it makes a great deal of sense purposely to make some space for ourselves so that we can recharge and replenish our mental, emotional and physical batteries.

left REGULAR PAMPERING SESSIONS, IN A SPA OR AT HOME, IS A GREAT AID TO RELAXATION AND DE-STRESSING.

Melting Stress: The Importance of Massage

Massage is one of the most relaxing and enjoyable treatments available. As with so many 'hands-on' therapies, the relaxation we experience as a result of a massage when our muscles have been tense and tight or generally stiff and painful is immediate.

If we are feeling especially fraught and tense, there is a great deal to be said for simply booking a massage treatment. After all, when we seem to be hemmed in on all sides, knowing that no one will be able to get to us while we are stretched out on the massage couch is a comforting, relaxing thought in itself.

If booking in for a regular full-body massage is too time-consuming or too pricey, you should at least consider having a weekly neck-and-shoulder treatment, as many stress-related problems, such as tension headaches, back pain and migraines, are aggravated by persistent – or severe – tension in the neck and shoulders.

Do not forget that you can also benefit from the relaxing and stress-busting effects of massage by literally taking the matter into your own hands and giving yourself a treatment once a week. The face, shoulders, hands and feet are all easy to reach and can benefit significantly from self-massage.

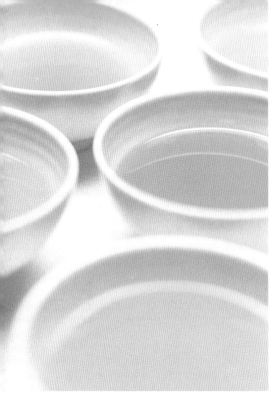

The Face

1 Having first warmed a small quantity of oil or gel in the palms of your hands, start with the delicate skin of the neck. Take care when working on the skin of the neck, making sure that you always use a light touch in order to avoid stretching or pulling the delicate skin around this area.

2 Massage the neck by moving from one side to the other, using light, upward-stroking movements: ideally, one hand should follow the action of the other in a continuous, rhythmical way. Continue with these movements for about three minutes.

3 Place your thumbs on the area just beneath your chin and put the balls of your fingers above. Slowly work your way outwards, using a pinching movement, until you reach the earlobes; you should be able to cover the whole distance in four pinching movements. You should then repeat the sequence ten times.

4 Next take the two first fingers of each hand and, starting near the nose, use small pressing movements to work your way slowly along the cheekbones. Use the balls of your fingers, making gentle and regular press-and-release movements until you get to the area of your jaw-bone joint (often called the TMJ joint, for short). Repeat this movement ten times, working from the original starting point each time.

5 Gently massaging the delicate skin around the eyes is an excellent way of adding essential moisture. By stimulating a more efficient flow of lymphatic fluid, it also encourages the drainage of accumulated fluid and toxins. Start at the outer edge of the bony eye socket, using the ball of your third finger on each hand to apply a firm and gentle pressure, working on the lower half of the eye socket and moving inwards and upwards past the nose to the eyebrow, and then back to the original starting point at the outer edge of the eye. Aim to repeat this circular motion ten times, remembering never to use dragging or pulling movements, and making sure that the pressure remains rhythmical, light and firm throughout.

above USE A SUITABLE OIL WHEN YOU ARE MASSAGING TO AVOID PULLING OR DRAGGING. right A FACIAL MASSAGE CAN BE PROFOUNDLY SOOTHING AT THE END OF A BUSY DAY.

Self-Massage Techniques

If you want to get the most from your self-massage, it is very important to use the correct type of oil; this will ensure that gliding movements travel smoothly across the skin without pulling or dragging it – especially important for delicate areas like the face and neck.

Use a special facial-massage gel or simple almond, olive or jojoba oil for massaging the face. The overall routine can take anything up to half an hour – or more, depending on how many areas you want to concentrate on – so ideally you should work in a comfortable chair. Most important of all, make the atmosphere of the room you intend to use as relaxing and soothing as possible. It should be warm and cosy, while candles and music can also help to create a sensuously pleasing atmosphere.

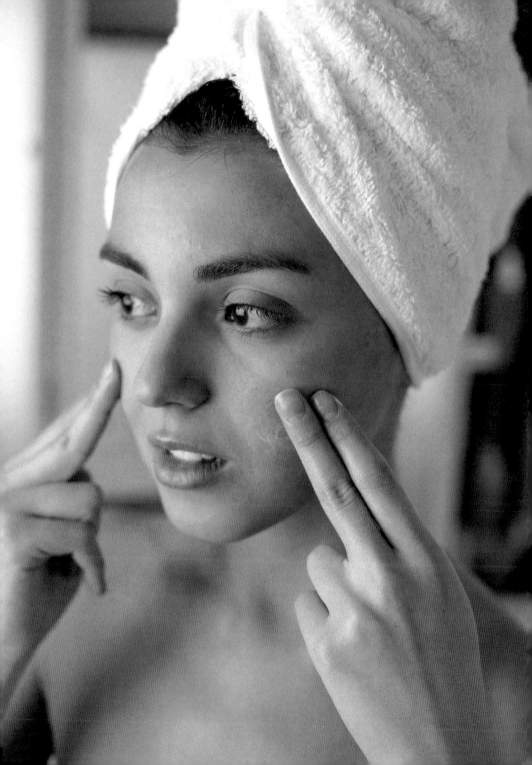

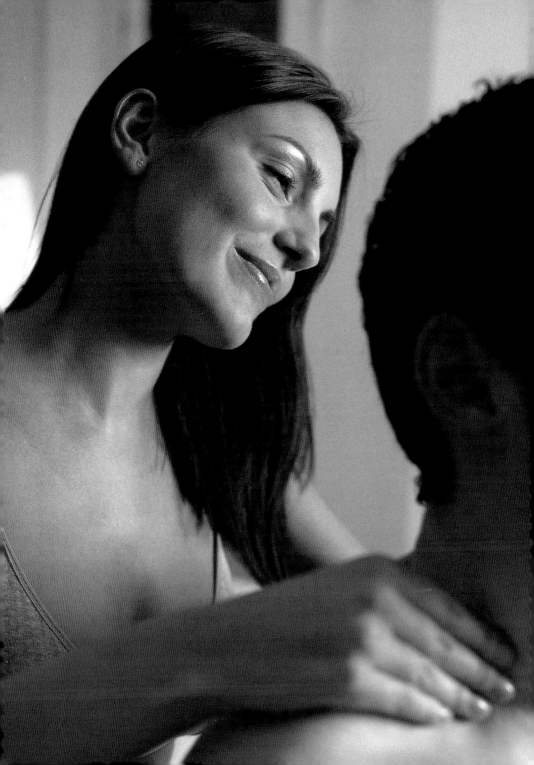

The Shoulders

1 Begin at the front, placing the two first fingers of each hand underneath the inner area of the collarbone at the base of the neck. Work outwards towards the shoulder joint with a light press-and-release movement; it should be possible to cover the distance in about four moves. Once you have reached the outer area of the shoulder joint, return to the original position and start again. Repeat the movement five times.

2 Work the back of the left shoulder using the three middle fingers of your right hand. Massage the large triangular-shaped muscle that lies at the back of the shoulder area, making rhythmical, circular movements, working inwards from the outer edge of the shoulder towards the spine. Use a sufficiently firm pressure to release the tension that so commonly builds up in this area. Spend as long as you feel you need to on the left shoulder before turning your attention to the right shoulder and working it in the same way, but with the three middle fingers of the left hand.

The Hands

1 With your thumb on top and index finger underneath, move rhythmically along each finger, working in an upward direction from the base of each finger to its tip. Start on the left hand, using your right thumb and index finger to work along the thumb, and then treating each finger in turn until you reach the little finger. Repeat this three times on each hand before loosening up the palm of the left hand by massaging it with your right thumb in a circular movement. Do the same with your right hand, then finish off by using the three middle fingers of the right hand to loosen up the back of the left hand, using small, rhythmical movements and working from the base of the fingers to the wrist. Repeat the process on the right hand.

The Feet

We can hold a surprisingly large amount of stress and tension in our feet – as we do in our hands – without being aware of it. Our hands and feet are both areas that tend only to attract our attention when they show signs of discomfort or are actually painful; otherwise they are often neglected. Paying attention to our feet by giving them a relaxing, moisturizing massage can pay great dividends, however, because we are likely to experience a profound sense of relaxation after working on our feet. For an especially reviving session, make sure you address any rough areas with an exfoliator before you start your massage.

1 Massage the whole of each sole first, using firm, rhythmical, circular movements. Only move on to the upper part of the foot when the soles of your feet feel thoroughly relaxed. Use the ball of the thumb and move in small, circular movements from the toes, up the foot and to the ankle.

left THE NECK AND SHOULDERS ARE A COMMON SEAT OF TENSION. below TARGET HOT-SPOTS IN THE SOLES OF YOUR FEET TO EASE ACHES AND PAINS AND IMPROVE CIRCULATION.

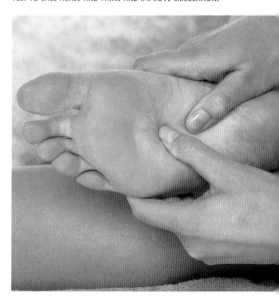

Energy Boost: Home Hydrotherapy

An accumulation of negative stress can leave us feeling sluggish, lacklustre and fatigued. And the effect will be exaggerated by a build-up of toxic waste in the tissues of the body – the result of poor eating and drinking habits, and a sedentary lifestyle (whether because of the pressure of stress or as a matter of choice). In such a situation, one of the best ways to give our systems a much-needed boost is to set to work immediately on stimulating a more efficient flow of lymphatic fluid, while we improve our eating and drinking habits. We can do this very easily for ourselves at home by establishing a regular combined routine of simple hydrotherapy and skin brushing.

Dry-Skin Brushing

We are dependent on the efficient flow of lymphatic fluid through our system to eliminate toxins, transport nutrients to our tissues, and basically to make sure that our immune system works at peak efficiency. If we adopt a regime that encourages good lymphatic drainage, we should find that fatigue becomes less of a problem and that premature ageing, which is connected to cell degeneration, is more likely to be postponed. In addition, there should be a reduced tendency to develop cellulite (the 'orange-peel' deposits that have a maddening tendency to develop on our buttocks and thighs).

Dry-skin brushing is claimed to be one of the most effective and direct methods we have at our disposal for stimulating the efficient flow of lymphatic fluid. All we need is a firm, natural-bristle brush.

- Adopt a 'hands-on' approach and dry-skin brush every day, either before showering in the morning or before bathing at night.
- Move upwards with large sweeping movements from the feet, up the front and backs of the legs, paying particular attention to the thighs and buttocks.
- Use firm, but not excessive, pressure and always avoid brushing any areas of broken veins or inflamed or broken skin.

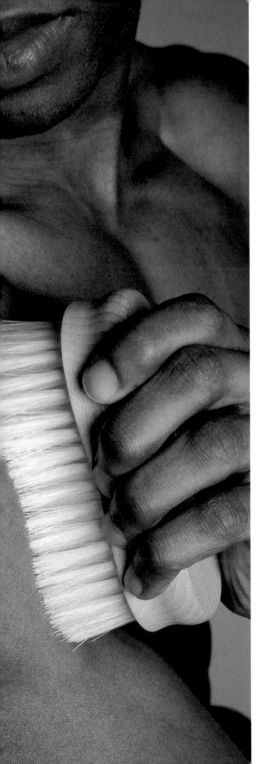

left DRY-SKIN BRUSHING IS SIMPLE TO DO BUT CAN STIMULATE A MORE EFFICIENT FLOW OF LYMPHATIC FLUID.

- When brushing the upper body, work in either a downwards or an upwards direction, using large, smooth movements, always towards the heart.
- There is no need to go into overdrive with dry-skin brushing: one regular session a day should be sufficient to stimulate the circulation and get lymphatic fluid moving more efficiently.

Simple Hydrotherapy Techniques

Regular hydrotherapy has a reputation for stimulating a sense of mental, emotional and physical wellbeing and vitality. It also appears to improve the cosmetic appearance of the skin, gives us greater protection against developing recurrent minor infections and boosts circulation. In addition, it stimulates the kidneys, bowels and lungs to function more efficiently, thereby encouraging an enhanced elimination of toxins.

Hydrotherapy treatments have been offered in European spa resorts for many years; they involve extremely high-pressure water jets being directed at specific parts of the body in order to stimulate circulation. It is possible to enjoy some of the benefits of hydrotherapy at home, however, with the use of nothing more sophisticated than a basic hand-held shower attachment.

NB *Anyone who is generally in good health and free from any chronic medical condition can explore home hydrotherapy without a qualm. If you are in any doubt at all about whether you should experiment with hydrotherapy, or if you suffer from angina, heart disease, psoriasis, eczema, varicose veins or varicose ulcers, please seek a professional medical opinion first.*

- To gain maximum benefits from a hydrotherapy session, have a skin-brushing session before you start. Then begin by taking a soothing shower that thoroughly warms up your body. Follow it with a refreshing cold shower, which should last about 20 seconds.

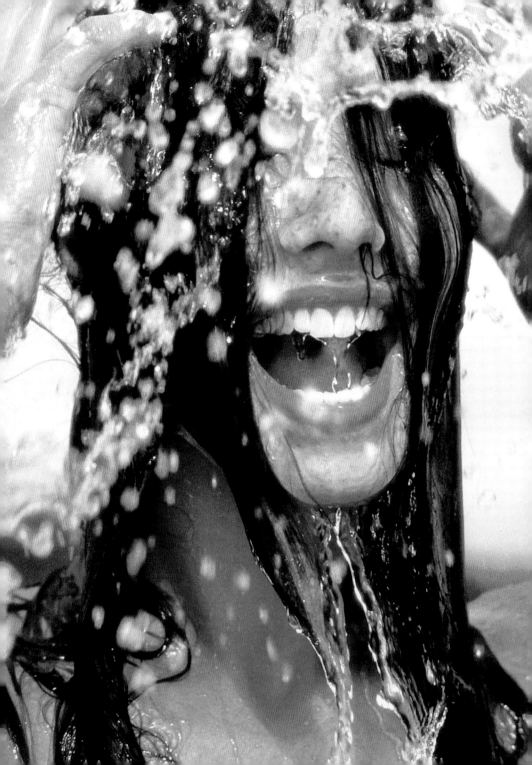

- After that, switch back to warm, then once you feel comfortably warm, have another quick burst of cold to finish.
- Do not worry if a 20-second cold shower feels too long at first; build up the length of the cold session slowly over time. Remember that this section is about health-giving, pleasurable experiences that we should really look forward to enjoying; there is little to be gained from something that makes you grit your teeth. If, on the other hand, 20 seconds feels fine, do keep in mind that it is possible to overdo things. It is, for instance, positively inadvisable to spend more than 30 seconds in a cold shower.
- Avoid starting with a cold shower, especially if you are already feeling chilled. To gain the maximum benefits, always warm up first.
- A short blast of cold water can help to tone up areas that are showing signs of poor, or sagging, skin tone. Areas that commonly benefit from specific attention include the thighs, upper arms and breasts.
- At the end of a hydrotherapy session, let the skin dry naturally in a steady, warm temperature rather than vigorously towel-drying the whole body for the sake of speed.

Scented Solutions: Aromatherapy Treats

Aromatherapy has an established reputation as an important complementary therapy, one that can stimulate a powerful sense of emotional, mental and physical wellbeing and balance. The basic tools of this therapy – highly concentrated essential oils – can be used in a variety of ways, depending both on our individual preferences and on practical limitations. Generally speaking, essential oils can be:

- Vaporized and inhaled
- Added in special blends to a carrier oil and used for massage
- Added to the bathwater to create a relaxing, invigorating or sensual bathing experience

In a stress-busting campaign, aromatherapy is one of the most practical and pleasurable tools we have at our disposal to help us unwind and relax. In order for essential oils to be vaporized, they need first to be mixed in water. To make a massage oil, by contrast, drop the various essential oils into a clean glass bottle (coloured rather than clear glass if you intend to store the oil), add a carrier oil (such as almond), then shake well to mix the contents thoroughly – and remember to shake the bottle again before you use it to agitate the contents. The effect the massage oil will have is determined by the individual properties of the various oils you have combined. The following blends of essential oils can be used either to stir your senses, or to help you switch off.

left and below WATER CAN HAVE AN ENERGIZING EFFECT WHEN USED IN A SHOWER (HIGH-PRESSURE OR NOT) BUT HAS SOOTHING PROPERTIES IN THE BATHTUB.

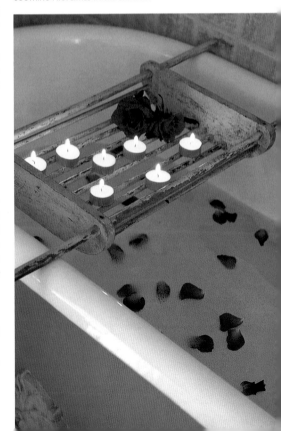

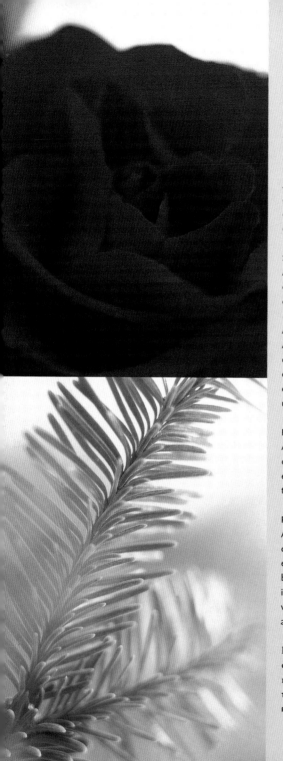

STRESS-BUSTING MASSAGE BLEND

Add eight drops of bergamot essential oil, three drops of clary sage essential oil, three drops of neroli essential oil and five drops of frankincense essential oil to 50 ml of carrier oil (either almond or unrefined sunflower oil).

UPLIFTING MASSAGE BLEND

Add four drops of lemon essential oil, eight drops of coriander essential oil, four drops of neroli essential oil and three drops of ylang ylang essential oil to 50 ml of carrier oil.

SLEEP-INDUCING MASSAGE BLEND

Add 12 drops of lavender essential oil, eight drops of neroli essential oil and five drops of rose essential oil to 50 ml of carrier oil.

ANXIETY-RELIEVING BLEND

Add six drops of juniper essential oil, three drops of rose otto essential oil, five drops of cedarwood essential oil and five drops of sandalwood essential oil to 50 ml of carrier oil – either almond or unrefined sunflower oil.

HEADACHE RELIEVING BLEND

Add two drops of peppermint essential oil, five drops of lavender essential oil and five drops of eucalyptus essential oil to a cream or gel base. Apply a little to the back of the neck and to the temples.

REVIVING VAPORIZING BLEND

Add five drops of cypress essential oil, five drops of pine essential oil and ten drops of rosemary essential oil to 100 ml of water in a dark glass bottle. Shake well to mix the liquid and then pour it into the well of a purpose-built essential-oil vaporizer. Use this blend whenever the going feels as though it is getting too tough.

left ESSENTIAL OIL OF ROSE IS SUPREMELY UPLIFTING AND CALMING, WHILE OIL OF ROSEMARY HAS A REVIVING EFFECT. right VAPORIZING ESSENTIAL OILS IS A SIMPLE WAY TO BRING THEIR MOOD-BALANCING AND DE-STRESSING PROPERTIES INTO THE HOME OR WORKPLACE.

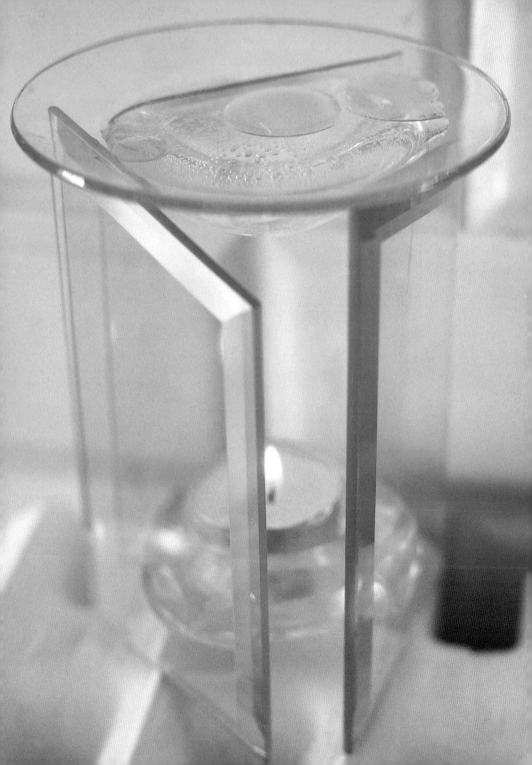

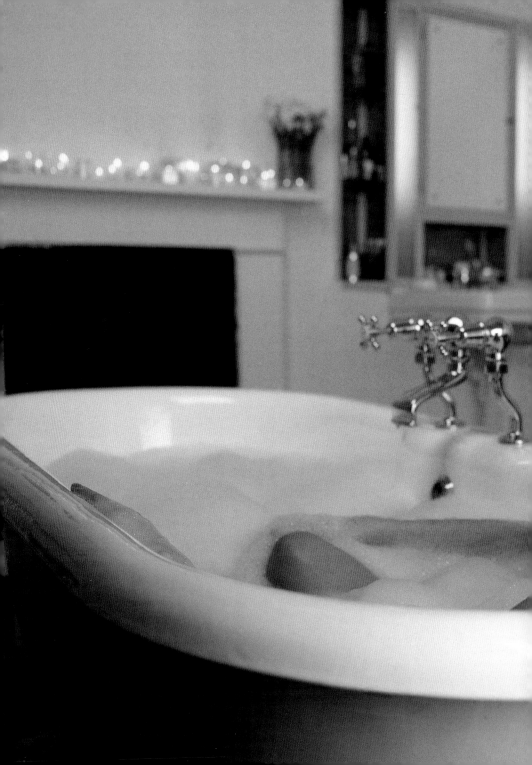

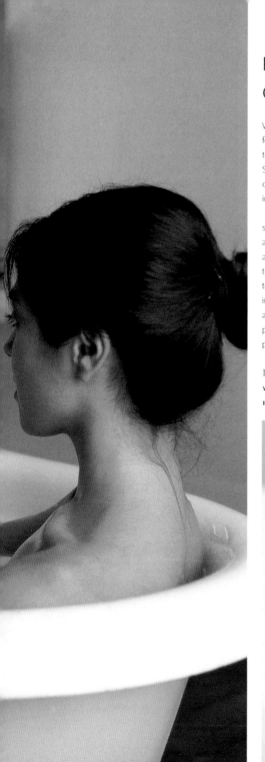

Blissful Bathing:
Creating a Home Spa

We all need a retreat to which we can retire when we feel strung up or stressed out. Which room we choose to turn into our stress-proof sanctuary is really up to us. Some people may instinctively feel that they want to concentrate on their bedroom, while others may have imaginative plans for a tranquillity-inducing study.

However, because the bathroom is already a space that is conducive to privacy, sensual pleasure and relaxation, it also provides great scope as a sanctuary. It makes sense, then, to spend some time thinking about how to make this room as pleasurable to use as possible. The following suggestions may inspire you, but let your own imagination roam freely and widely as well – it will guide you to create a safe, personalized haven where you can feel entirely protected from the rigours of life.

left FLICKERING CANDLE-LIGHT IN THE BATHROOM IS A SIMPLE WAY TO CREATE A RELAXING ATMOSPHERE. below HERBAL INFUSIONS ADDED TO THE BATHWATER CAN HELP US TO UNWIND.

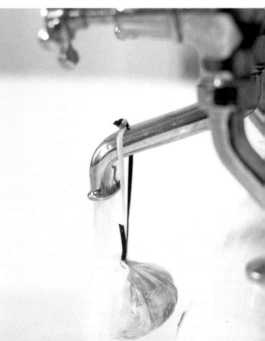

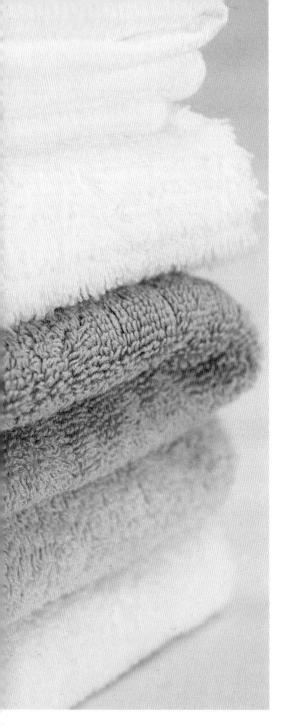

- Consider softening the ambient lighting by using candles creatively. You can buy all sorts of ingenious holders today: a 'chandelier du bain' is perhaps one of the most decadent – a detachable fixture for the side of the bath with a candle-holder on one side, and on the other a small, flat, circular disc that is the perfect size for a champagne glass.

- When selecting candles, opt for those that are scented with essential oils, which will delight two senses at once.

- Remember that if you are fully to unwind, you need to treat your visual sense as much as possible. When you decorate your bathroom, choose colour combinations that instinctively appeal to you, however unorthodox they might seem to others. Add stencilled patterns or hang pictures, photographs or prints that you love (but remember that steamy environments can be damaging to some media).

- On a practical note, make sure that your bathroom is well heated. There is nothing so unrelaxing when we need to unwind and let go of the accumulated tensions of the day as feeling chilly.

- Invest in some good-quality, soft towels that feel soothing to the touch. Bathrobes, too, should be of a sufficiently good-quality cotton that they never feel harsh against the skin.

- It is amazing to discover how therapeutic a little judicious 'clutter clearing' can be. Throw away anything that is not serving any positive purpose.

- If you need a tension-busting, sleep-inducing soak, try adding two or three handfuls of Dead Sea Salts to a warm bath, together with five drops of lavender or sandalwood essential oil, and bask in the warm water for ten minutes or so before showering off the salts with soothing warm water. Wrap yourself in a warm bathrobe, sip a cup of camomile tea, switch off the light, retire under the bedclothes as soon as possible and relax.

left CHOOSE COLOURS FOR YOUR BATHROOM ACCESSORIES THAT YOU FEEL MIGHT HAVE A THERAPEUTIC EFFECT. right AS WELL AS ENCOURAGING DETOXIFICATION, DEAD SEA SALTS CAN HAVE A POWERFUL STRESS-REDUCING ACTION.

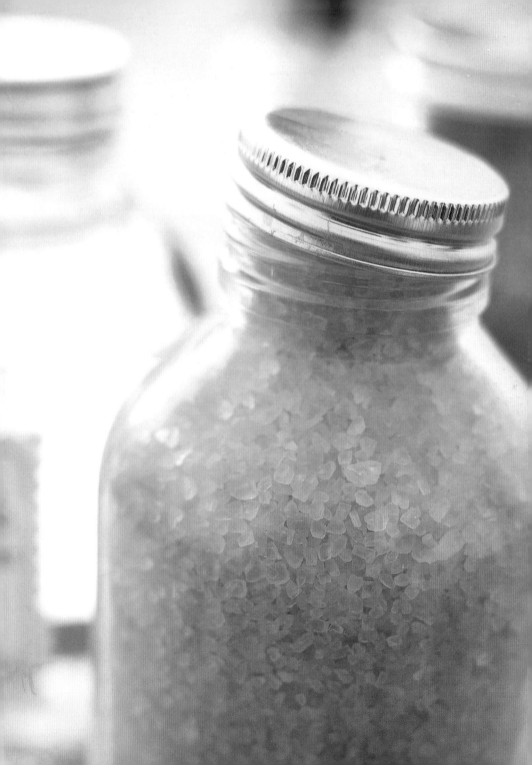

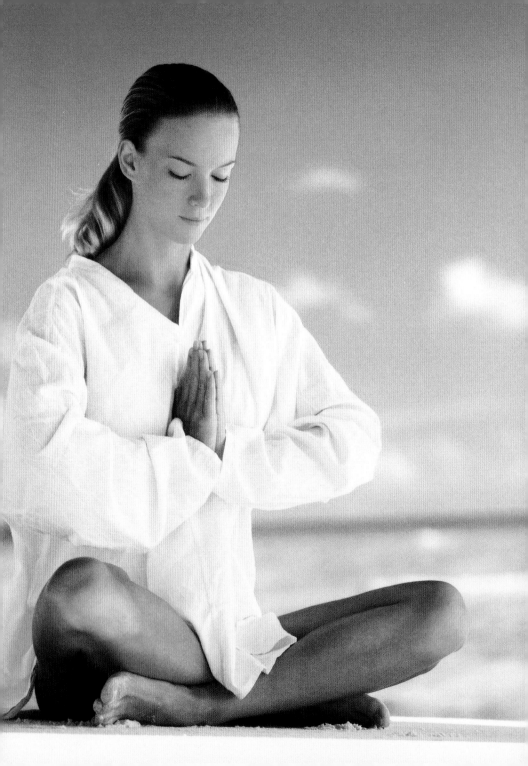

Rebalance: Fast-Track Alternative Solutions To Stress-Related Problems

THIS SECTION ADOPTS A QUICK-FIX APPROACH TO TREATING SOME OF THE COMMON CONDITIONS THAT AMBUSH US WHEN WE HAVE BEEN UNDER THE STRAIN OF NEGATIVE STRESS FOR TOO LONG, AS WELL AS OFFERING SOME ADDITIONAL ADVICE WITH REGARD TO LIFESTYLE CHOICES – DESIGNED TO EASE THE PRESSURE WHEN THE GOING GETS TOO TOUGH. THE SELF-HELP MEASURES DESCRIBED ARE ROOTED, ON THE WHOLE, IN PRACTICAL HOMEOPATHY, HERBALISM AND AROMATHERAPY.

Only measures known to be non-addictive have been recommended, and largely only those things unlikely to cause side effects. If you are in any doubt about the suitability of any treatment because you are already taking prescription medication, do not hesitate to seek professional medical advice – from your own GP, or local pharmacist, or from an alternative or complementary therapist.

If, having adopted one of the following measures, you experience only a short-lived improvement in your general wellbeing or in relation to one specific problem, do not immediately assume that further improvement will not be possible. Instead seek professional advice from an alternative therapist working in the relevant field, outlining what has happened during, and in response to, self-treatment.

left RELAXATION TECHNIQUES CAN BE EFFECTIVE IN HELPING US TO SWITCH OFF FROM ANXIOUS THOUGHT PATTERNS – EVEN IF ONLY FOR A WHILE.

Natural Treatments for Anxiety

Anxiety is a multifaceted condition that can, therefore, be characterized by an extremely broad variety of symptoms. Everyone is probably familiar with 'butterflies', that fluttering sensation in our stomachs that occurs in anticipation of an exciting or demanding occasion, but which tends to disappear as soon as the event is over and we are able to unwind and relax. Even as a minor symptom, though, butterflies serve to demonstrate how anxiety or 'nerves' can affect us.

At the other extreme, the severe end of the anxiety spectrum, major anxiety symptoms can – disturbingly – appear out of nowhere, with no obvious trigger. Full-blown anxiety attacks can affect our whole system; we feel dizzy, breathless, sick and engulfed by panic. If left unattended, severe anxiety can make even day-to-day living an uphill struggle, for small problems can become exaggerated through anxiety, and if these are allowed to undermine our confidence, as if eating away at our inner strength, anxiety can sometimes develop into real phobia.

Someone who is experiencing moderately severe anxiety symptoms because of escalating levels of stress at work or at home stands somewhere

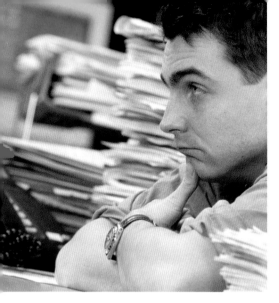

practitioner may also be able to provide you with the emotional support that you need in the first instance to use conventional medication.

While the severity of certain features may vary, the following are common symptoms of anxiety:

- Palpitations (consciousness of an irregular or rapid heartbeat)
- Nausea
- Perspiration
- Diarrhoea
- Light-headedness
- Tingling in the hands and arms
- Rapid, shallow breathing
- Dry mouth
- Cramping pains in the stomach and abdomen
- Disturbed sleep
- Shaking and trembling in the muscles

Breathing

above ANXIETY LEVELS CAN ESCALATE AT WORK IF WE FEEL THAT WE ARE BEING ASKED TO HIT IMPOSSIBLE TARGETS. right DIAPHRAGMATIC BREATHING TECHNIQUES HELP US TO FOCUS THE MIND AND RELAX THE BODY.

between these two extremes, ideally placed to benefit from the self-help strategies suggested below. These can make a huge difference, supporting us through the turbulence of anxiety caused by a temporary stress overload. Once these measures begin to take effect, we will find that a sort of breathing space will appear. It is at this point that we will be able to take stock of the situation and try to find ways of managing stress levels more effectively.

If, on the other hand, you feel as though the situation has moved beyond self-help measures, your symptoms having become more severe, try not to dismiss out of hand alternative or complementary therapies per se. On the contrary, it is always worth consulting an alternative medical practitioner, such as a homeopath or Western medical herbalist, because these therapists work with medicines that not only ease the symptoms of anxiety very effectively but also avoid the dependence problems that are known to arise from the prolonged use of conventional medication, such as tranquillizers.

Moreover, it is worth bearing in mind that if the situation is especially severe, an alternative medical

If we want to tame feelings of panic and anxiety, one of the most important things we can do is to learn how to regulate our breathing. Our natural tendency, when we are under great stress and pressure, and if we are not advised otherwise, is to breathe rapidly and shallowly from our upper chests. This actually makes the situation worse, because this pattern of breathing triggers an imbalance in our blood gases (oxygen and carbon dioxide) that makes us feel even more tense and anxious.

On the other hand, if we know how to use our breathing patterns to induce a relaxed, clear-headed state, we need never – even when we are under pressure – feel as out of control again.

This form of breathing, called diaphragmatic breathing, is the sort of breath-control technique that is taught in yoga. It has been developed from the simple idea that much of the time most of us neglect to use the lower part of our lungs when we breathe, and that this grows much worse when we are under stress – the very time, ironically, when we need to use our full lung capacity to calm ourselves down.

In order to learn how to tap into the benefits of diaphragmatic breathing, begin by observing how you breathe usually. Sit in a straight-backed chair and

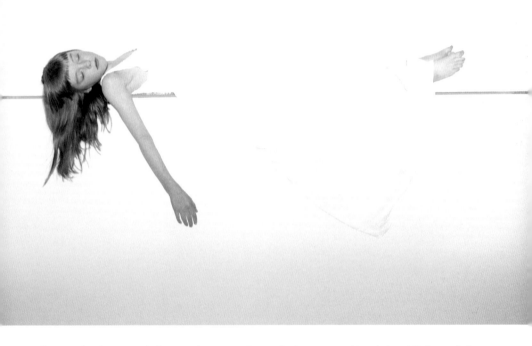

place one hand on your belly somewhere around your navel. At this point you should make a conscious effort not to change the way you are breathing; just observe what is happening. It is more than likely that your hand is barely moving. Now take a long, deep breath that fills your lungs slowly from the top all the way down to the base. As your lungs fully inflate with air you will find that your hand rises. As you breathe out, and as your lungs empty from the base to the top, your hand will move back to its original position. Take five more breaths in this way, concentrating on – and taking note in your mind of – the sensations evoked by the technique. Once you become fully familiar with what this technique feels like, you will be able to use it discreetly whenever things are becoming tense and fraught, to restore some sense of clear-headed calm.

If, when you use this technique initially, you feel a little light-headed, do not panic. Just breathe normally for a few breaths and try again. Aim for regular and unforced breaths, inhaling and exhaling for the same length of time on each breath.

Diet

There are certain foods and drinks that actively contribute to an established state of anxiety – and heighten its degree of intensity – making the situation worse. Drinks that make us feel very jittery and tense include strong tea, coffee, caffeinated colas and fizzy 'energy' formulas that provide us with a liberal dose of caffeine. Foodwise, anything containing hefty amounts of sugar, and chocolate in any form, can make us feel 'wired-up' and moody.

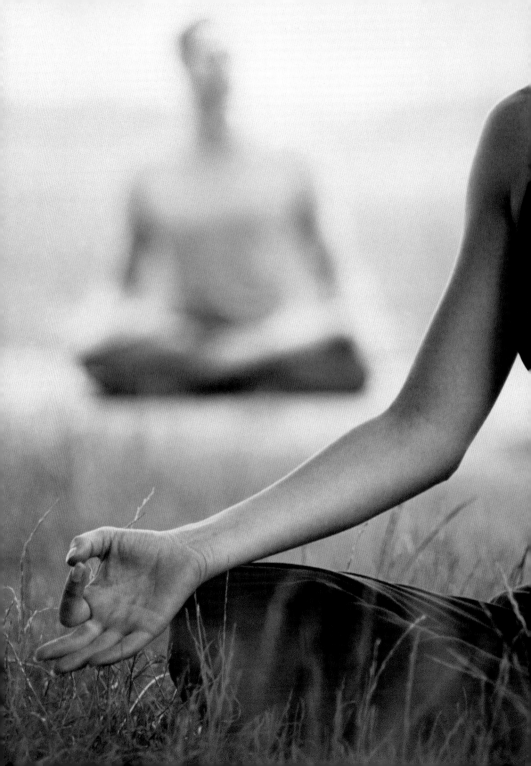

We should opt instead for calming foods that provide a sustained energy release: wholemeal bread, fresh fruit (especially bananas, because of their tryptophan content), dairy foods, avocados and lettuce, for example. As far as drinks are concerned, camomile tea is one of the most soothing; drink it whenever you are feeling uptight and nervous. You should also avoid having long gaps between meals if you are stressed: having a snack every two hours will help to keep your blood-sugar levels stable.

Exercise

Those of us who have overwhelmingly sedentary, high-pressure lives are far more likely to suffer from pent-up anxiety and mental and physical tension than those of us who exercise regularly. If you generally take very little exercise, you should try to begin giving your heart, lungs and muscles the thorough workout they need as soon as possible. It is vital to choose an activity that suits your temperament; otherwise you will get bored, and boredom is one of the greatest stressors known to man or woman. Swimming, walking and cycling are all excellent options, while yoga, T'ai chi and Qi gong are more relaxation-oriented systems. It is also important to remember to build up slowly, rather than overdoing things in the first flush of enthusiasm.

Essential Supplements

The full spectrum of B vitamins are known to support a stressed nervous system, so taking a good-quality vitamin-B complex will provide long-term benefits.

Kava kava is gaining a reputation as an effective alternative to conventional tranquillizers; apparently it is free of the acknowledged dependency problems associated with the benzodiazepine tranquillizers. But if you are already taking conventional tranquillizers or antidepressants, do not take kava kava: the interaction of the two is potentially problematic.

left TIME FOR EXERCISE AND RELAXATION NEEDS TO BE BUILT INTO A DEMANDING LIFESTYLE. right RESCUE REMEDY IS AN EXCELLENT NON-ADDICTIVE AID TO RELAXATION.

Aromatherapy

Enjoy an anxiety-busting soak by adding five or six drops of essential oil to a bathtub filled with warm water: bergamot, lavender, clary sage and ylang ylang are all known for their relaxing properties. Use them individually or in combination – your sense of smell should delight in the scent. For maximum therapeutic effect, drip the oil into the water after you have turned off the taps (faucets); otherwise the essential oils will evaporate while the water is still running.

Make your own massage oil by adding two or three drops of an essential oil for every 5 ml of carrier oil: camomile, geranium, bergamot and clary sage are all good for defusing anxiety.

Alternatively, vaporize any of these essential oils in a custom-made vaporizer; or add a drop or two to a tissue and inhale the extract whenever you are feeling on edge.

Flower Essences

Whenever the early warning signals of stress and anxiety appear, try to keep these unwelcome feelings at bay by taking a few drops of Bach Rescue Remedy. The small dropper-bottles fit easily into a handbag – or even a pocket. Either place a few drops under the tongue or add the recommended number of drops to a small glass of water or fruit juice and sip the tincture as often as you feel the need.

Herbal Help

When you sense an imminent invasion of feelings of tension and anxiety, sipping an infusion of soothing herbs can be very effective: try camomile, valerian or lime flower. Choose carefully, bearing in mind that if you are to gain the maximum benefit from a herbal infusion, its taste should be appealing – in the same way that any essential oils you use should delight your sense of smell. Change your choice of infusion regularly, too, because taking any single herb for too long is not advisable. Valerian, for example, taken infrequently, in small doses, can do a great deal to calm the mind and encourage a state of relaxation, but taken as a matter of routine it can contribute to – or aggravate – problems with palpitations, headaches and muscle spasms.

Homeopathic Remedies

Aconite Upsetting news may result in episodes of anxiety characterized by feelings of terror and panic that dishearten you abruptly; these tend to be worse at night, accompanied by severe palpitations and physical and mental restlessness. Such anxiety may respond very well to a few doses of aconite.

Gelsemium Slow-developing anxiety that tends to escalate in anticipation of a particularly stressful event (giving a major presentation at work, for instance) may be considerably relieved by treatment with gelsemium. Indications that this remedy is needed are becoming withdrawn and irritable (until the event is over), and suffering from persistent, painless diarrhoea and recurrent tension headaches that feel as if the forehead has been restricted by a tight band.

Arsenicum album This can be very effective in the treatment of anxiety that occurs when someone is pushing himself or herself to meet unreasonably high, perfectionist standards – and if other characteristic features are present. These include disturbed sleep – waking at 2 am feeling extremely anxious, restless and chilly – and a tendency to become obsessive when under pressure.

Phosphorus This can be very helpful for those who are normally outgoing, energetic and confident, but who experience 'free-floating' feelings of anxiety when exhausted. This leads to a state of anxiety that is unconnected to any specific issue, but which seems to be able to attach itself to anything that is currently happening. People who need this remedy are very sensitive to the feelings and moods of others, and can pick up an atmosphere without really trying.

Natural Treatments for Depression

Depression effectively provides a mirror image of anxiety. In fact, the two conditions often occur side by side, so that it is very rare to meet someone who has experienced anxiety who has not also felt low from time to time. Equally, the severity of both conditions can vary greatly.

In the same way that an episode of anxiety can be brief or extend over a long period, depression can either trigger very minor symptoms or be a life-constricting experience. We can feel mildly 'blue' for no obvious reason or sense a definite awareness of being jaded and low in response to a specific upsetting event. Depression problems can also result from the cumulative effect of a combination of stresses that hit us at a time when we do not feel resilient enough to deal with them.

The measures that follow can be of great benefit to someone suffering from depression that has occurred in response to a specific stressful event or a series of minor problems that mount up, causing an excessive negative stress load. In other words, this section is about self-help treatment for the 'blues'; it does not attempt to deal with full-blown, established clinical depression. Alternative and complementary therapies can still be of great value with regard to this latter condition, but, for the most successful outcome to emerge, a trained practitioner needs to be involved. This is partly because of the complex nature of depression, but more to do with the adverse interaction of medicines. While not a problem with regard to homeopathic treatment, this can be a complication in relation to Western medical and traditional Chinese herbal medicines, a complication that needs to be addressed responsibly by a trained practitioner in either therapy. So if you are already taking conventional medication, always seek advice before supplementing it with a herbal preparation.

right **ALTERNATIVE AND COMPLEMENTARY THERAPIES HAVE A GREAT DEAL TO CONTRIBUTE IN THE TREATMENT OF MILD TO MODERATE DEPRESSION.**

Mild to moderate depression can be characterized by any of the following symptoms:

- Disturbed sleep patterns, with a tendency to wake early feeling anxious and/or depressed
- Loss of appetite
- Poor concentration
- Lack of motivation
- Fatigue
- Mood swings
- Lowered libido
- Recurrent negative thought patterns
- Hyperventilation and/or palpitations

There are specific life events that can leave us vulnerable to feeling low and 'blue'; any of the following are likely triggers:

- Pregnancy – the state itself and its aftermath
- Redundancy
- Dramatic changes in financial status
- Menopause – the change itself and the reality of the post-menopausal condition
- Bereavement
- Relationship breakdown

Exercise

Paradoxically, although the last thing we want to do when we are feeling low is to take exercise, it is one of the most effective tools we have at our disposal for lifting our mood. Regular aerobic exercise has been shown to stimulate the production in our bodies of feelgood chemicals called endorphins (responsible for the 'high' experienced by runners and cyclists). Because we breathe more deeply and rhythmically when we exercise, regular exercise also boosts the elimination and removal of toxic waste from our bodies, and effective and efficient detoxifying in this way can play an important part in making us feel more mentally and physically energized and alert.

If we suffer from mild to moderate depression, then, which will almost certainly leave us feeling constantly exhausted and lacking in motivation and concentration, exercise is crucial. When we exercise, however, we should make sure that we do not get so breathless that we are gasping for air; this would indicate anaerobic activity, which cancels out the benefits of aerobic exercise.

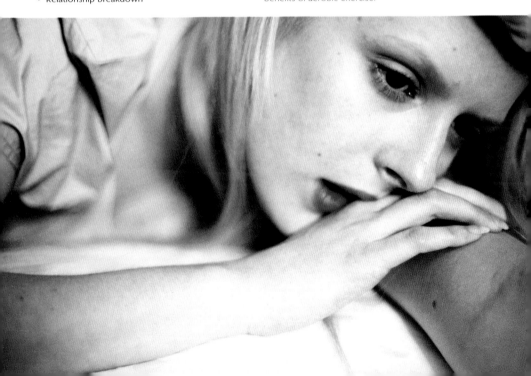

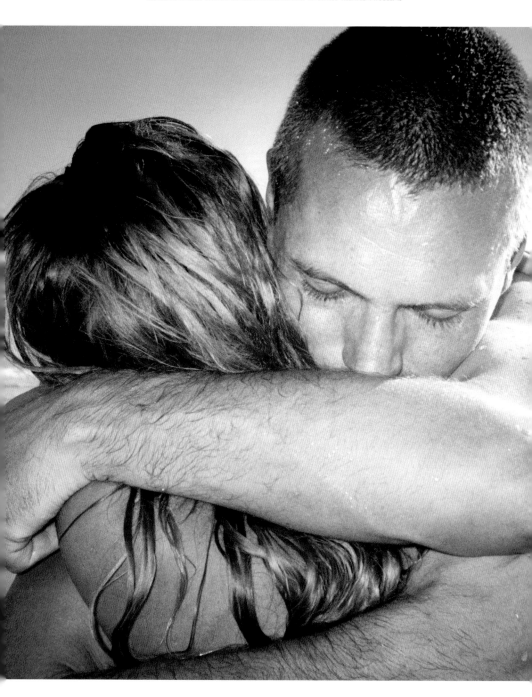

Talking

If you have felt low for some time and there have been no signs of the depression lifting, it may be very therapeutic to talk through some of the major issues of concern, but you must feel that you are talking within the boundaries of a safe space. You could talk frankly to a close friend, family member, partner or colleague. Bear in mind, though, that those who are close to you may be too emotionally involved to be able to listen uncritically and objectively to what you have to say, especially if you are being unnervingly honest. What is crucial is that you choose someone who you feel you can trust completely.

This may mean that it could be more helpful to step outside your immediate environment, to talk over the main issues with a trained counsellor or psychotherapist. A professional listener will be able to take the necessary objective stance and will interpret what you are saying with the benefit of a trained perspective and experience of similar situations. As a consequence, such a listener is likely not only to be able to facilitate the exploration of certain issues (which might result in emotional insights), but will also be able to support you through the process.

NB *As depression is more often than not accompanied by anxiety, it will probably be useful to look again at the general self-help part of the anxiety section (page 99).*

Essential Supplements

Often when we feel low our eating patterns suffer as a direct consequence. This can be partly due to the loss of appetite that is a common and characteristic feature of depression. Moreover, the lack of interest and motivation that can also go hand in hand with feeling low is likely to compound the problem.

If such a situation develops, it is advisable to take a good-quality multivitamin and multimineral supplement to make sure that at least the basic nutritional needs of the body are being met during times of emotional stress.

If negative stress levels have been especially high for an extended period of time, it is worth taking a course of vitamin-B complex in order to give the nervous system a boost. The B vitamin folate, especially, has been shown to play a crucial role in the alleviation of depressed feelings. In fact, if you are deficient in B12, this will leave you prone to suffer from feelings of depression.

Vitamin E balances dopamine levels, which not only regulate mood but can also provide an important buffer against the stress response. The recommended dose is 3–4 mg per day; foods rich in vitamin E include wheatgerm, nuts, unrefined oils, such as sunflower oil, and foods made from wholegrain ingredients.

Ginseng seems to be able to stabilize the levels of neurotransmitters in the brain, and therefore has a balancing effect on moods. It should help us to fight the depressive effects of long-term negative stress.

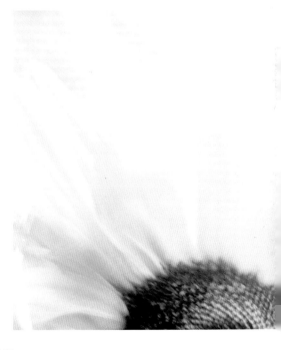

left **WE OFTEN NEED EMOTIONAL SUPPORT WHEN WE ARE FEELING BLUE, BUT ARE UNABLE TO SHOW IT.** right **THE OIL EXTRACTED FROM SUNFLOWERS IS A RICH SOURCE OF VITAMIN E.**

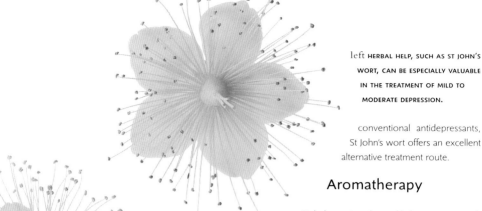

conventional antidepressants, St John's wort offers an excellent alternative treatment route.

Aromatherapy

To help you to relax and balance your mood, add camomile, clary sage, lavender, marjoram or ylang ylang essential oils – singly or in combination – to the bathwater. Bear in mind, though, when you are using essential oils, that they are extremely concentrated and should be used very sparingly. Four or five drops is all you need to create a mood-balancing bathing experience.

Homeopathic Remedies

Depression arising from the cumulative effect of emotional strain or grief often responds very well to natrum mur. Those who need this particular remedy have a tendency to keep a stiff upper lip; find talking about their feelings very painful and difficult; and seem to obtain no relief from bursting into tears on a sympathetic shoulder – perhaps even finding it makes matters worse. Such people studiously avoid lively or sympathetic company, and view peace and quiet as definitely desirable.

Pulsatilla can be regarded as being appropriate for someone displaying the opposite symptoms of the 'blues' from those that will respond well to natrum mur. People will respond well to this remedy if they are unashamedly weepy and tend to cry over nothing, and if crying makes them feel much more cheerful and generally better. The positive results of this good cry will be enhanced if there is a sympathetic shoulder upon which to cry, so someone in need of pulsatilla is likely to try to avoid being alone, actively seeking out company instead. Someone suffering from temporary depression premenstrually, or during or after pregnancy, could benefit from pulsatilla.

Herbal Help

The use of the herbal medicine St John's wort (also known as hypericum) has recently attracted much publicity in relation to its potential use as an effective, natural antidepressant. Witness the fact that in Germany today it has been calculated that someone diagnosed as suffering from mild to moderate depression is ten times more likely to be prescribed St John's wort than Prozac or any other type of selective serotonin reuptake inhibitor (SSRI) antidepressant.

Recently, however, one potential drawback of St John's wort has been uncovered: the possible negative interaction of this herbal medicine with a specific range of conventional medicines. These include antiepileptic medication; drugs that are used to minimize the likelihood of rejection following an organ transplant; medication used to treat asthma or bronchitis (theophylline, specifically); drugs used to treat heart problems; some anticlotting agents; some migraine treatments; the contraceptive pill; medication used to treat HIV; and some other prescription antidepressants.

St John's wort is most useful when mild to moderate depression has been diagnosed and there is no previous history of taking antidepressant medication. In such a context, and particularly if there are any reservations about potential side effects of

Feelings of apathy, indifference and depression that result from a condition of severe emotional, mental and physical exhaustion can be perked up considerably by a few doses of sepia. While I have treated plenty of men very effectively with sepia, women do seem to respond especially well to this remedy, especially if they are suffering from depression following childbirth, or as a result of going through the menopause. Flagging libido and a total lack of interest in sex (both connected to overwhelming stress levels) are also strong indicators of the need for this remedy.

Agitated, anxious depression that is much worse when the sufferer is alone at night may respond well to arsenicum album. Sleep disturbance will be a particular problem here, the marked tendency being to wake at around 2 am, before tossing and turning for the rest of the night. Those needing arsenicum album may be hit by depression simply because they fail to meet the unrealistically high, unachievable standards they set for themselves. Appearing to be 'driven', such people are likely to be difficult to work or live with because of their fussy, fidgety moods and critical intolerance of themselves and anyone around them.

Natural Treatments for Tension Headaches

Recurrent tension headaches that extend from the base of the skull to the front of the head are an obvious sign that stress levels are getting out of control. There are certain widely acknowledged offenders that can trigger or aggravate these draining headaches. Identifying which of these are relevant in a particular situation can be tremendously beneficial, because armed with this knowledge we can take positive action to change our situation for the better, and limit the frequency and severity of attacks.

Common factors that can trigger tension headaches include any of the following:
- Muscle tension in the jaw, neck and shoulders
- An excessive intake of coffee, alcohol or pain-killers containing codeine

- An irregular or infrequent intake of food
- Mediocre working conditions – a VDU screen positioned at the wrong angle, for example, or a chair of an inappropriate height
- Changes in eyesight that have not been registered; having regular eye tests every two years is essential once we reach the age of 40
- Low-grade dehydration
- Postural problems

Of course, if you start to suffer from regular and severe headaches for no obvious reason, it is sensible to consult your GP to have the problem checked. If the examinations or tests do not reveal a pathological cause, you can take further comfort from the fact that there are positive steps you can take that will reduce your stress load generally and deal with the specific aspects of your lifestyle that may be burdening you.

below **AN EXCESSIVE INTAKE OF CAFFEINE CAN BE RESPONSIBLE FOR TRIGGERING SEVERE HEADACHES.**

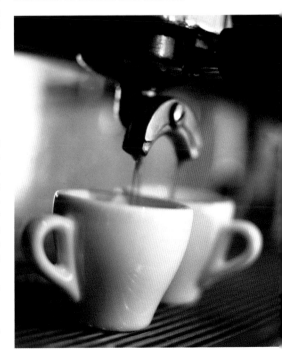

Massage

If muscle tension in the neck and shoulders is an insistent, well-established problem, it is well worth having a regular neck, shoulder and back massage. Quite apart from being blissfully relaxing, this will have a directly beneficial effect – loosening bunched-up muscles in the neck and shoulders and improving the blood supply to the area.

Chiropractic and Osteopathy

It may be helpful, for more severe and established neck and shoulder problems, to seek treatment from a chiropractor or osteopath; either will be well qualified to rectify any mechanical irregularities that might be triggering persistent headaches.

Diet

If your intake of caffeine or alcohol has been steadily rising in response to an increasing and unusual amount of stress and pressure, follow the advice on kicking the caffeine habit and kicking the alcohol habit (see pages 61 and 62).

Lighting

Check that the lighting at work is not responsible for – or contributing to – your headache. Replace any flickering fluorescent lights and ensure that your work space is sufficiently well lit, because eye strain will only aggravate your problem.

Bed

If your neck stiffens up as you sleep and you feel uncomfortable and unrelaxed when you wake, it is time to buy some new pillows. There are a huge number to choose from, stuffed with natural or synthetic materials, so seek expert advice on the advantages of the different types before you invest. Comfortable enough to help you enjoy a sound night's sleep, your pillows should also be firm enough to give the neck and head adequate support.

right EASE CONGESTION BY INHALING THE AROMATIC STEAM OF DROPS OF PEPPERMINT ESSENTIAL OIL DILUTED IN HOT WATER.

Relax

If, when you are under stress, you clench your jaw, this may contribute to tension problems in the large muscles of the neck and shoulders. Established and severe problems with jaw tension can also result in teeth-grinding while you are asleep. To check this tendency, make a point of relaxing the muscles of the face and jaw when you feel you are under pressure; consciously relax both shoulders – you should find that they drop away from your ears by about 5 cm (at least 1 in) as you let go of the tension, and relax your arms and hands. If you find it difficult to do this – or to retain any degree of relaxation – it may be helpful to have lessons from an Alexander Technique teacher (see page 79).

Aromatherapy

Tension headaches can be eased by diluting about four drops of peppermint oil in a tablespoon of carrier oil and rubbing it gently along the hairline and forehead using a cotton-wool bud (Q-Tip). If sinus congestion is adding to your headache problems, you may find it more effective to inhale: either add a few drops of peppermint essential oil to a bowl of hot water and inhale the steam, or place a couple of drops on a tissue or handkerchief and, holding it at least 5 cm (1 in) away from your nose to prevent your skin from coming into direct contact with the essential oil, take a sniff from time to time to clear your head and blocked sinuses.

Putting a couple of drops of clary sage, diluted in a carrier oil as described above, on a cotton-wool bud (Q-Tip) and running it around the hairline and across the forehead can soothe tension headaches that appear and increase in severity in the days immediately prior to a menstrual period. Alternatively, you may prefer to add five drops of essential oil to your bathwater for a long, warm and fragrant soak. While it is advisable to use only clary sage during the days running up to and on the first day of your period, you may like to add soothing lavender at other times.

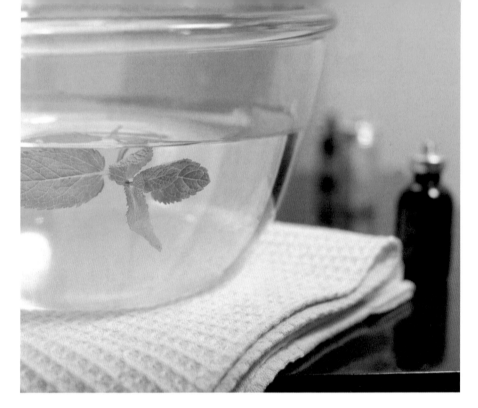

Herbal Help

Sip a cup of dandelion tea to ease a headache that appears after a period of excessive eating and drinking.

Drinking an infusion of lime flower, valerian or lemon verbena will be soothing if you are suffering from a tension headache that has taken a hold after a period of extreme pressure. You can use ready-prepared teabags or loose, dried herbs. If you are using the latter, pour a cup of boiling water on to a teaspoonful of your chosen herb and leave it to infuse for 15–20 minutes before you strain it.

Homeopathic Remedies

Tension headaches that are triggered by dehydration, and made much worse by the slightest movement, may respond very well to bryonia. Someone requiring this remedy will report that the pain characteristically begins above the left eye before radiating to the nape of the neck. When the headache begins to throb, the entire scalp may also feel sensitive to the slightest touch.

'Toxic' headaches that follow on from a disastrous cocktail of late nights, excessive alcohol, too many cigarettes, junk food and extreme pressure at work almost always respond magically to nux vomica, too. Just like a hangover, this type of headache feels particularly awful when you first wake in the morning and is especially severe at the back of the head. Not surprisingly, anyone suffering from this type of headache is extremely irritable and 'short-fused', and craves peace and quiet.

Tension headaches that have been aggravated by skipping meals because of extreme stress and pressure may be improved by sulphur. When this remedy is needed, there is a heavy, throbbing sensation at the crown of the head, and it feels as though the brain is being squeezed in a vice. General sensations of dizziness and light-headedness caused by low blood-sugar levels become more severe if the sufferer bends forward.

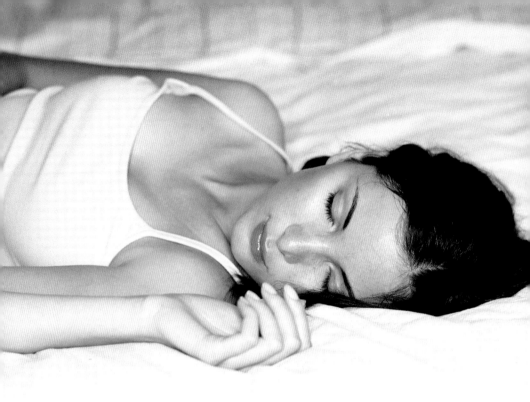

Natural Treatments for Insomnia

Few things are as exhausting and frustrating as being unable to get a refreshing, sound night's sleep when we need it. Moreover, enjoying a full night's rest is essential if we want to achieve and maintain high-quality health. This is because it is when we sleep that all our organs have a much-needed chance to rest and replenish themselves, and when the subconscious is able to maintain our mental and emotional health by working safely through all the material accumulated in the mind during the day – in the form of dreams. Sleep deprivation, on the other hand, has been proven to have a negative effect on the functioning of our immune system, leaving us prone to recurrent infections and a general sense of feeling burnt out and run down.

An overload of negative stress is one of sound sleep's greatest enemies, because a build-up of mental, emotional and physical tension does not set us up well for a relaxed rest. The physical reaction to stress or pressure – the fight-or-flight mechanism (see page 19) – floods our systems with adrenaline to enable us to take prompt and decisive action.

It is easy to see how, if this is happening regularly on a daily basis, without any physical outlet being provided for the adrenaline that is whizzing around our bodies, we are bound to feel agitated and wakeful by the time we try to go to sleep. This is what causes the unpleasant sensation of feeling completely physically exhausted at bedtime, and yet being unable to get our minds to switch off enough to let us fall asleep.

Any, or a combination, of the following factors can also trigger bouts of sleeplessness:

- Premenstrual syndrome
- Menopause
- An overactive thyroid gland
- Anxiety
- Depression
- Chronic fatigue syndrome
- Post-traumatic stress disorder
- Bereavement
- Caring for a young baby
- Nursing a sick relative

Sleep disturbance can vary in character and intensity. Some of us may find that although we go to sleep perfectly easily, we wake after only an hour or so feeling ready to get up. Others may find it incredibly difficult to calm down and go to sleep. Others again may doze fitfully throughout the night without achieving any real depth of sleep, so that, when morning comes, they are likely to feel totally unrefreshed and less than ready to spring out of bed.

How much sleep each of us needs to function at an optimum level will vary from person to person, so there are no hard-and-fast rules. The chances are that each of us knows instinctively how many hours' rest we need each night.

If your sleep pattern is disturbed for more than a brief period, you may – and frequently will – begin to display any of the following symptoms:

- Irritability
- Poor memory
- Diminished concentration
- Excitability and impatience
- Recurrent infections, such as sore throats, colds and coughs

Your Bedroom

Make sure that your bedroom is conducive to good, sound sleep. Essential features of a bedroom that promotes tranquillity include:

- Curtains or blinds that are heavy enough to block out light adequately, but not so heavy that they make waking up difficult

- Good ventilation, so that the room is neither too stuffy nor too chilly
- As quiet a room as possible. If this is difficult to achieve, it may be worth considering installing double-glazing in order more effectively to minimize excess noise
- A good mattress. It is easy to forget that mattresses have to be replaced regularly; on no account sleep on the same mattress for more than ten years. When choosing a replacement, look for one that provides firm support without feeling hard: rest should be a comfortable experience

Switching Off

If you want to sleep soundly you must steadfastly resist the temptation to work until just before you go to bed, however tempting it may be at times of high pressure. This is because, if you do, your mind will be still mulling over problems and working on finding solutions just when it needs to be relaxed and letting go of worries as a prelude to sleep. Instead, try to make a point of doing something relaxing for an hour or two before preparing to sleep.

There are lots of practical, pleasurable ways of encouraging the mind and body to slow down and switch off. You may find that some of the following inspire you: choose whichever you feel suits your temperament, in order to induce a state of relaxation:

- Soaking in warm – but not too hot – scented bathwater
- Listening to the radio
- Playing a favourite piece of music that makes you feel positive and relaxed
- Listening to an audio book
- Meditating or working through a guided-relaxation technique
- Sipping a soothing, warm drink
- Making love

Avoid using a stiff drink to induce a drowsy state because although, in the short term, alcohol acts as a relaxant, its long-term effects actually have a disruptive effect on sleep patterns and adversely affect the rest achieved; alcohol-induced sleep is poor-quality rest and therefore less refreshing. Too much alcohol can also make us feel less than invigorated in the morning.

Avoid eating heavy or indigestible meals late at night, as this can trigger digestive discomfort that can in turn contribute to poor-quality, fitful sleep.

Releasing Tension

If you toss and turn at night because of muscle tension and aches and pains, you should consider a two-pronged plan of action. Have a regular, full-body aromatherapy massage to help your body unwind, and make a point of taking some sort of exercise at least three times a week: either rhythmic, aerobic activity, which gets the circulation moving and conditions the large muscle groups, or a more relaxing system of movement that elongates and relaxes the muscles – yoga or T'ai chi, perhaps. If you are feeling tense, the breath control that is integral

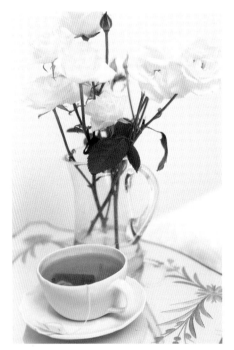

to these latter will prove an added benefit because it can be used to induce a state of relaxation.

Essential Supplements

See the discussion of kava kava in Nourish (page 70).

Aromatherapy

To create a sleep-inducing massage oil, blend three drops of the essential oils of lavender, camomile and mandarin in two teaspoons of carrier oil. This should only be used on adults.

Herbal Help

Avena sativa compound, which comes in liquid form in an easy-to-use dropper-bottle, is an especially effective alternative to conventional sleeping pills. It is a combination of sleep-inducing herbs – including valerian, passionflower, hops and oats – and a homeopathic preparation of coffee. About 20 or 30 drops in a small glass of water should be taken before you go to bed.

Alternatively, moderate or infrequent problems with insomnia may be alleviated by drinking an infusion of camomile. If you are using fresh herbs, add a teaspoonful to a cup of boiling water, cover, and leave it to infuse for 15 minutes before straining and sipping the liquid – either as a relaxing early evening drink, or at bedtime.

Homeopathic Remedies

Anxious insomnia resulting in a positive phobia about going to bed can be eased considerably by lachesis. A tendency for sleep problems to appear, or become aggravated, in the days leading up to a menstrual period (when mood swings are also likely to be especially marked) would serve to confirm the

left SOOTHING CAMOMILE TEA CAN HELP US TO SWITCH OFF AT THE END OF A BUSY DAY. right A HERBAL TINCTURE LIKE AVENA SATIVA THAT CONTAINS PASSIONFLOWER CAN HELP GET A TEMPORARILY DISTURBED SLEEP PATTERN BACK ON TRACK.

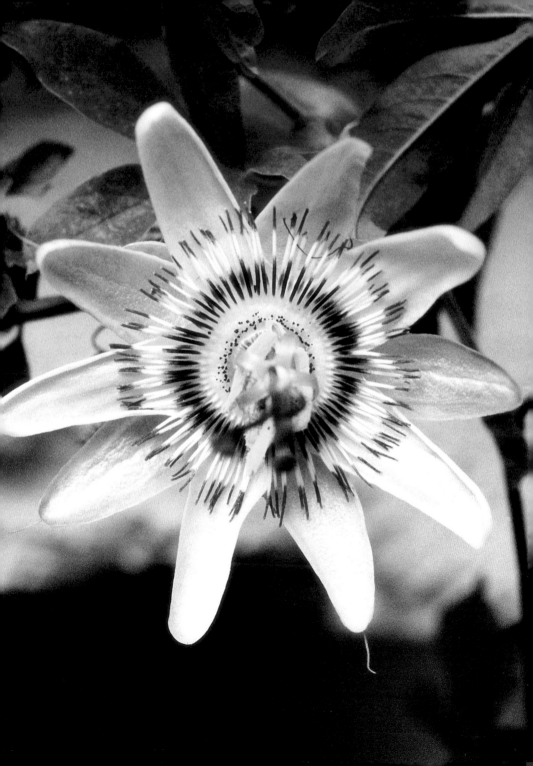

need for this homeopathic remedy. Someone who experiences a distressing, jolting sensation or a feeling of suffocation as they drift off to sleep will also benefit from lachesis.

Perfectionists who push themselves too far for too long, and who suffer as a result from problems with anxiety and insomnia may respond well to arsenicum album. Characteristically, when this remedy is needed there is a tendency to go to bed mentally and physically exhausted and to fall asleep quite quickly, only to wake again at 2 am. Once awake, the mind is beset by anxious thoughts whirling around, which often make going back to sleep impossible. If, in addition, a habit has developed of getting up to make a soothing warm drink rather than continuing to toss and turn, this remedy is definitely worth a try.

Sound sleep patterns that have been shot to pieces by too much pressure, alcohol, coffee and other caffeinated drinks should be treated with nux vomica. Someone who responds well to this remedy tosses and turns all night, before finally falling soundly asleep only an hour or two before the alarm goes off. Hangover-type headaches, nausea, constipation and severe irritability and impatience are all symptoms that can benefit from this remedy. Compulsive partygoers should never be without nux vomica.

Sleep that is disturbed following the shock of receiving upsetting news may respond very well to ignatia. When this remedy is needed the picture is unmistakable: rapid mood swings are common and there is a strong tendency, when overtired, to feel weepy or irritable. Falling asleep is likely to be very problematic, and there will be persistent yawning and muscular twitching.

Natural Treatments for Irritable Bowel Syndrome

Our digestive systems tend to act as barometers of stress levels. As a practitioner, I have yet to meet the patient who is suffering from excessive levels of negative stress and who does not have some sort of digestive discomfort. Most of the common

problems can be discussed under the general umbrella heading of irritable bowel syndrome (IBS), although symptoms of stress-related digestive problems can include any of a variety of complaints, including:

• Persistent indigestion
• Heartburn
• Loss of appetite
• Abdominal bloating
• Cramps
• Alternating diarrhoea and constipation

Irritable bowel syndrome is a common problem and is recognized as being a condition that is likely to afflict those adversely affected by a stress-filled life. For those unfortunate enough to suffer from IBS, therefore, learning effective stress management should be high on the priority list. There are, as well, other self-help measures that can make an important and positive difference.

Diet

Certain foods are known to aggravate IBS problems. Common culprits include: wheat (in items such as bread, pasta, cereals and sauces); sugar in the form of fizzy drinks, cakes, cookies and chocolate, together with 'hidden' sugars that come incorporated in baked beans, soups and processed foods; pulses, beans, Brussels sprouts; and products made from cows' milk. If you suspect that one of these items may be behind your digestive problems, try an elimination programme. Avoid this particular item for a month and monitor any changes in the function of your digestive tract. If you notice an obvious improvement, reintroduce the eliminated item and watch to see how your body reacts. If troubles return, eliminate the item again. If, as a consequence of this, there is a further improvement, the chances are that you do have a sensitivity to this item so should try to avoid it as much as possible.

If you discover that you have a number of food sensitivities it is well worth consulting a homeopathic practitioner. He or she will probably prescribe a treatment to regulate your digestive tract. This may take some time, but the overall health benefits of treatment can be impressively wide-ranging, and if it means that an overreaction is less likely to occur in the long term, this time will seem insignificant.

Constipation problems are frequently just the result of simple, low-grade dehydration, so make a point of drinking quantities of still mineral or filtered tap water daily. Steer clear of fizzy mineral waters, particularly if abdominal bloating is a problem, because these can considerably aggravate any tendency to flatulence.

Avoid, or at least radically cut down your intake of, tea, coffee, colas and alcohol, as these drinks have a reputation for irritating the digestive tract. Remember, too, that cigarettes have an irritating effect on the lining of the stomach, which means that regular smoking can worsen any problems with heartburn and indigestion.

Eating a healthy amount of fibre-rich food is critical for promoting smooth digestive function, although an overenthusiastic intake of fibre can exacerbate problems with diarrhoea. If frequent bouts of diarrhoea seem always to be followed by a few days of constipation, so that a cyclical pattern is established, eating a substantial quantity of vegetables is to be recommended – lightly steamed to make them more easily digestible. Home-made soups, too, can add extra fibre to the diet in a non-irritating way.

High-fat foods should be treated with extreme caution because they are especially difficult to digest. Avoid foods, then, that are recognized to be high in saturated fat – full-fat cheese, red meat, butter and cream – and make a point of trimming off the skin from chicken before you eat it because, while the meat has a relatively low fat content, a great deal of fat is stored in the skin. Equally, rather than battered, deep-fried fish, it is much better to choose grilled or baked fish, cooked with a little cold-pressed, virgin olive oil.

Essential Supplements

Aloe vera has acquired a reputation for soothing the digestive tract and gently encouraging regular bowel movement, with none of the dependency problems and overenthusiastic action that are associated with conventional laxatives. It is also a suitable supplement to take when you are suffering from a stomach bug because of its antiseptic and immune-system-enhancing properties. Whether you choose to drink the slightly bitter aloe vera juice or take tablets or capsules is a matter of personal preference; the benefits will be the same.

Aromatherapy

You can help ease a feeling of general queasiness by gently massaging the skin just above the rib cage with a soothing blend of essential oils: two drops of black pepper, camomile, peppermint, ginger and mandarin essential oils added to two teaspoons of carrier oil. This blend should be avoided, however, if the feelings of nausea and queasiness are symptoms of pregnancy.

below **ALOE VERA APPEARS TO HAVE AN EXTREMELY SOOTHING EFFECT ON THE DIGESTIVE TRACT.**

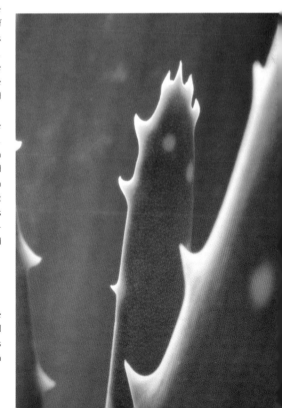

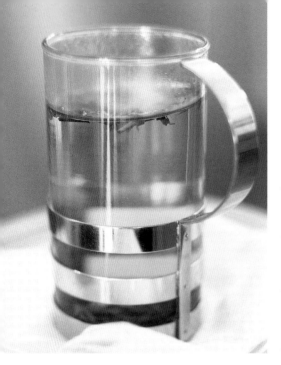

left **AN INFUSION OF CAMOMILE TEA, WITH A LITTLE GRATED GINGER, MAKES A SOOTHING DRINK WHEN WE FEEL QUEASY.**

Symptoms of digestive problems that are made noticeably worse by a combination of high levels of nervous tension and a high intake of sugar may be eased considerably by arg nit. The need for this remedy is characterized by an abundance of noisy wind that seems determined to travel both upwards and downwards. When diarrhoea and constipation are present, they are usually accompanied by lots of abdominal swelling and bloating. When stressed or agitated, someone in need of this remedy will also become 'hyper' and overtalkative.

IBS problems that emerge in tense, nervous people who feel compelled to live in the fast lane can often be banished by a few doses of nux vomica. Digestive pains, exacerbated by an overreliance on coffee, alcohol, cigarettes and painkillers, will seem to be further intensified by jarring movement. And if severe or persistent constipation is present, there is a tendency to feel headachy, hungover, irritable and grouchy.

Herbal Help

Occasional indigestion and overacidity can be soothed almost instantaneously by a warm drink of slippery elm. Stir two heaped teaspoonfuls of slippery elm powder into a cup of warm milk and take morning and evening until the stomach feels more settled.

Trapped wind and queasy indigestion can be considerably relieved by sipping an infusion of peppermint or camomile tea – livened up by a little freshly grated ginger.

Homeopathic Remedies

A few doses of lycopodium will dispel digestive uneasiness that is accompanied by lots of gurgling, burping and flatulence. A tendency to recurrent heartburn, with occasional episodes of acid rising into the throat and an uncomfortable, alternating pattern of diarrhoea and constipation would confirm the choice of this remedy. Anticipation of emotional and mental strain – public speaking being a notable usher of extra negative stress – will often trigger, or aggravate, all the symptoms for which this remedy is needed.

Natural Treatments for Recurrent Infections

Whether our immune system functions healthily and efficiently depends to a large degree on stress levels and how well they are managed. As a result, if we have been under excessive pressure that we have felt powerless to deal with for too long, it is very likely that we will begin to suffer from a succession of minor infections. If we become aware that we have been lurching from one cold to another, it is high time to examine how much pressure we have been under in recent months. If we realize that we have been stressed to the limit, it is the moment to take positive action and rebuild our body's defences.

Exercise

Moderate exercise has been shown to boost the efficient function of the immune system. Ideally, you should avoid anything that is overly taxing and competitive – training for, or running, half-marathons, for instance – because excessively demanding or punishing exercise has been shown to depress the immune system.

Enjoyable exercise, such as regular walking or non-competitive cycling, on the other hand, not only conditions the heart and lungs and does a great deal to keep us generally physically fit; it also helps to defuse stress. Alternatively, choosing a form of movement that combines muscle stretching with relaxation – yoga, for example – can give positive support to our mental, emotional and physical health. The stress-busting benefits that have been shown to flow from this sort of activity appear also to have a bolstering effect on immune-system performance.

Diet

What we choose to eat is known to have a profound effect on how efficiently our immune system performs. If we have been especially stressed and feel run down, increasing our intake of fresh, raw vegetables will be hugely beneficial – partly because of the antioxidant nutrients that yellow, orange, red and dark green fruit and vegetables have been shown to possess. We should, at the same time, make a point of minimizing our consumption of cigarettes, alcohol and foods and drinks saturated in sugar, as these actively depress the immune system.

Sleep

Endeavour to get plenty of good-quality, restful sleep because sleep deprivation has been proven to have an extremely negative effect on a number of levels simultaneously. Not only are we likely to feel irritable, woolly-headed, fatigued and less able to cope with pressure if we are unable to enjoy a good night's sleep each night; if we are deprived of sleep for some time, we will also find we become prone to minor infections. This is because it is only while we are

asleep that our immune system has the opportunity to rest and recharge. If we are under a great deal of stress, therefore, and we want to avoid feeling burnt out and run-down, getting a good eight hours' sleep a night should be high on our list of priorities. If the quality of our sleep has suffered because of excessive stress levels, the advice given in Natural Treatments for Insomnia (page 112) should prove helpful.

Essential Supplements

Vitamin C plays a crucial role in supporting our immune system when it has to fight infection. At the first sign of a sniffle, sore throat or feverishness, take 1 g of vitamin C (1,000 mg) a day. A slow-release formula is best for maximum impact and effectiveness because it will ensure that the benefits of the vitamin remain in the body for up to eight hours at a time. Alternatively, you could take one 250 mg tablet four times a day to achieve the same prolonged effect. Reduce the dose, however, if you experience any symptoms of acidity in the stomach or the slightest case of diarrhoea.

Garlic has an impressive reputation as a natural antiviral and antibacterial agent. It is difficult to eat

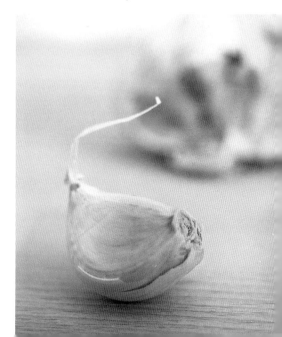

right GARLIC IS AN IMPRESSIVE ALLY IN ANY FIGHT AGAINST INFECTION – EASILY TAKEN IN CAPSULE FORM.

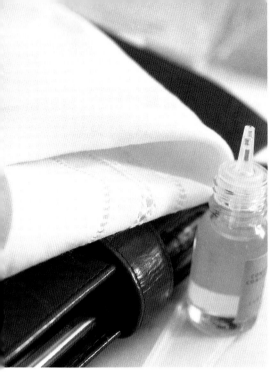

or sinus problems. Whether you choose to take the remedy as tablets or capsules, or as a liquid tincture or elixir, follow the dosage instructions supplied by the manufacturer. Most importantly, do not be tempted to take a daily maintenance dose of echinacea over the winter months. This particular herbal treatment's maximum benefit will be reaped only when it is taken in short courses – dealing with a specific infection.

Homeopathic Remedies

If symptoms of a minor infection are severe and have developed abruptly – especially after exposure to dry, cold winds, or getting generally chilled – a few doses of aconite may help. This is a fast-acting remedy that is especially effective in easing feverishness accompanied by sore eyes, nasal passages and throat. It is particularly appropriate for treating any minor infections that develop when the immune system has been suddenly depressed – after a shock or after hearing bad news, for instance.

If symptoms have progressed gradually and insidiously over a period of a few days, on the other hand, and there is a sense of feeling run down and exhausted, gelsemium would be a more suitable treatment. This remedy is indicated when someone is suffering flu-like muscle aches and chills that run up and down the spine. The nose is likely to feel persistently stuffed up and there may be an uncomfortable dryness in the throat with a loss of voice. Headaches are also considerably eased by this remedy, especially when it feels as though there is a tight band around the forehead.

If cold sores appear as a symptom of feeling run down, and there is a tendency to bottle up feelings and keep a 'stiff upper lip', natrum mur can help a great deal. When this remedy is needed, the general picture is one of dehydration: lips are generally sore and cracked (especially in the middle of the bottom lip) and the skin feels parched and tight when the person is in less than top form healthwise.

enough fresh garlic to secure its therapeutic effect, so taking it in concentrated tablet form tends to be more practical. Take a supplement that combines garlic with the antioxidant vitamins A, C and E for maximum infection-fighting power.

Aromatherapy

Adding five or six drops of lavender or tea tree essential oil to warm bathwater will provide you with an especially comforting soak.

The stuffy-headedness that is associated with a developing cold can be eased a great deal by inhaling a few drops of tea tree, eucalyptus or lavender essential oil from a handkerchief or tissue.

Herbal Help

When we develop signs of infection under stress, echinacea is one of the most effective immune-system boosters we can use. Take echinacea to shorten the duration of a cold and keep its complications at bay; or to promote a swift recovery from a sore throat, cough

Natural Treatments for Burnout

The term 'burnout', generally used to describe a state of profound emotional, mental and physical fatigue, really speaks for itself. Generally, burnout occurs in two different ways. It can either be the result of the cumulative effects of a stress-filled lifestyle that has gone on for too long, or it can develop from a particularly stressful or shocking life event that has proved too much for body, mind and emotions to cope with at that juncture.

Because burnout affects so many different aspects of our health at once, symptoms can be very general and broad-ranging and may include any, or any combination, of the following:

- An inability to concentrate
- Overwhelming fatigue
- Severe or unpredictable mood swings
- Recurrent minor infections
- Poor or disturbed sleep patterns
- Diminished levels of confidence
- Anxiety
- Depression
- An inability to switch off or relax
- Digestive problems, including indigestion, lack or loss of appetite, stomach acidity and/or alternating diarrhoea and constipation
- Generalized muscle stiffness, aches and pains
- Muscle weakness
- A general lack of motivation and focus

The advice that follows is likely to be of most benefit to those who are generally in sound good health, but who have found that a temporary crisis has depleted their energy levels and vitality completely. Those for whom stress management has been a long-term concern may need to seek professional advice and support to get them back on track. This could come from an alternative practitioner such as a homeopath, traditional Chinese therapist, Western medical herbalist, Ayurvedic specialist, reflexologist, masseur or cranial sacral therapist. It is also advisable to consult a GP.

It might sometimes be worth considering a more psychological approach, in which case consulting a stress counsellor or cognitive therapist would be the route to pursue. Cognitive therapy can be particularly liberating as it helps us to gain insights into patterns of behaviour that are preventing us from getting to grips with stress management. Identifying these patterns will move us to a position where we can begin to choose a different way to respond to the pressures and stresses in our lives (see page 107).

General Self-Help

Think about the foods and drinks to which you gravitate when you feel pressured and overwhelmed with stress. If you find that to try to keep up with the pace you turn to coffee, sugar, chocolate and alcohol, you will inadvertently and unfortunately be contributing to burnout. All these aggravate problems with mental and physical tiredness, jitteriness, disturbed sleep and mood swings. They also tend to place a toxic burden on the liver, so that if you rely too often and too much on these items, you are likely to look and feel lacklustre.

If we are genuinely determined to keep burnout at bay, we should make sure that as a matter of priority we practise relaxation techniques regularly. By enjoying regular, deep relaxation we are giving our minds, emotions and bodies a much-needed chance to relax and replenish. See Chapter Three (page 26) for advice on aids and suitable techniques, and on how to set about learning to relax.

Establish the boundaries you need to work within so as to remain productive and inspired, but protected from demands that heap excessive, draining burdens of pressure on you. This involves applying the skills described in Chapter Three (especially the practical strategies for de-stressing at work and at home, see pages 39 and 43). Once you have enjoyed the liberating benefits of effective delegation you will never look back.

An enjoyable, regular and appropriate exercise programme will play an essential role in promoting optimum balance and harmony on all levels – mental, emotional and physical – while also providing an important benefit in conditioning the immune system.

Feelings of tension and anxiety can be gently yet effectively banished by regular yoga or T'ai chi, while more vigorous exercise, like running or swimming, can help us to unwind at the end of a tough day.

Essential Supplements

Schisandra has been demonstrated to possess adaptogenic properties similar to those of ginseng. As a result, it can play an extremely positive role in supporting the body when it is confronted with an unusually high stress load. It appears to stimulate increased oxygen intake by the cells of our bodies, while also having properties that maximize concentration levels. Moreover, schisandra seems to have a beneficial effect in balancing mood swings, so that the irritability and anxiety that so often characterize burnout are likely to be less of a problem. The recommended daily dose for a course of treatment, taken in capsule form, is 250–500 mg.

When you are attempting to prevent the development of burnout symptoms, do not forget that the vitamins that make up B complex have a particularly important role to play in supporting our immune systems at times of protracted stress. To increase your intake of foods rich in vitamin B, choose wheatgerm, wholegrains, seafood, eggs, green, leafy vegetables and yeast extract.

Herbal Help

Whenever you are in need of a mental, emotional and physical energy boost make an infusion of the energy-balancing herbs and add it to a warm bath. To prepare a strong infusion, add three generous handfuls of dried peppermint or lavender to a medium-sized pan of cold water and leave the infusion to soak overnight, then bring it to the boil the following day. Once the liquid has reached boiling point, remove it from the heat and strain off the clarified liquid. Let the infusion cool before decanting it into a clean glass container that can be sealed with a tightly fitting lid. Whenever you are feeling tense, stressed and exhausted, add a generous amount of this infusion to your bathwater. All you need to do

then is lie back, relax and inhale deeply. If you have not used fresh herbs to scent your bathwater before, start with only a small amount.

If you have been under too much strain for too long, a tincture of wild oats can do a great deal to rebalance energy levels. It can also help to restore vitality if you are feeling very run down after a severe viral illness. Take eight to ten drops daily in a glass of water until energy levels are regained.

Homeopathic Remedies

Digestive problems that accompany burnout – flatulence, bloating, acidity and persistent indigestion – may respond very well to a few doses of lycopodium. The need for this remedy is indicated by diminished self-confidence and increased anxiety in response to an excess of negative stress.

Launching into a demanding physical training programme without proper preparation can result in physical burnout: the body feels bruised and sore and aches all over – making it impossible to be comfortable when trying to rest – and there is a pervading sense of exhaustion. These symptoms can be eased very quickly by a dose of arnica.

Those who become anxious and worn out as a result of pushing themselves to meet excessively punishing and overambitious standards should consider taking a few doses of arsenicum album. This remedy is indicated when there is a clear pattern of extreme physical and mental restlessness with a tendency to become obsessive when burnt out – in relation to exercise, irrational fears of illness and phobias about excessive cleanliness, for instance.

An occasional short course of nux vomica is a must for highly competitive overachievers who are hooked on stimulation of all kinds and find it almost impossible to switch off without alcohol or some kind of chemical assistance. Their coffee and alcohol intake will increase under pressure, and they are all too prone to become addicted to 'jogger's high' and the competitive aspect of exercise and sport.

right **IF YOU FEEL STRESSED AND HEMMED IN, A DOSE OF FRESH AIR IS A SIMPLE WAY OF CLEARING THE MIND.**

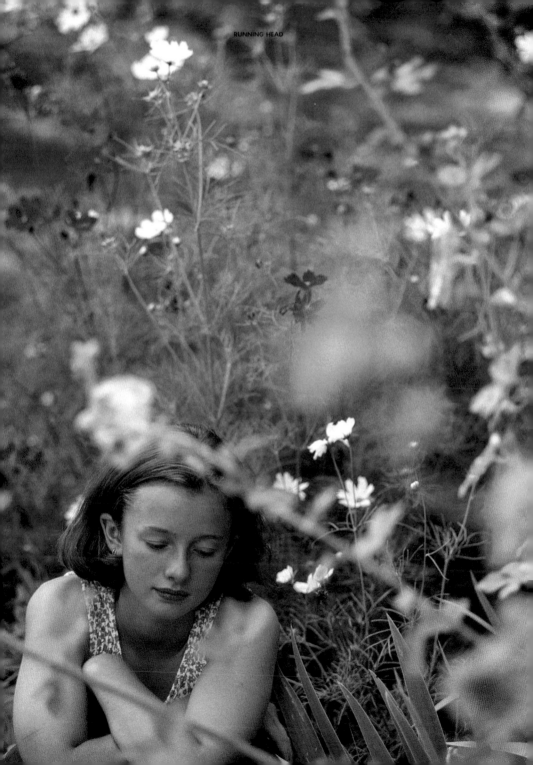

Recommended Reading and Address Book

Recommended Reading

Benson, Herbert MD, *Beyond the Relaxation Response*, Collins, 1985.

Benson, Herbert MD, *The Relaxation Response*, Collins, 1976.

Campsie, Jane, *De-Stress*, Murdoch Books, 2000.

Castro, Miranda, *Stress: Homeopathic Solutions for Emotional and Physical Stresses*, Macmillan, 1996.

Guiffre, Kenneth, MD, *The Care and Feeding of Your Brain: How Diet and Environment Affect What You Think and Feel*, Career Press, 1999.

Kenton, Leslie, *10 Day De-Stress Plan: Make Stress Work for You*, Random House, 1994.

Kirsta, Alix, *The Book of Stress Survival: How to Relax and Live Positively*, Gaia, 1986.

MacEoin, Beth, *Boost Your Immune System Naturally: Your Essential Guide to Fighting Infection and Nurturing Your Health*, Carlton, 2001.

MacEoin, Beth, *Natural Medicine: A Practical Guide to Family Health*, Bloomsbury, 1999.

Pfeiffer, Vera, *Stress Management*, Thorsons, 2001.

Selby, Anna, *Home Health Sanctuary: Weekend Plans to Detox, Relax and Energise*, Hamlyn, 2000.

Viagas, Belinda Grant, *Stress: Restoring Balance to Our Lives*, The Women's Press, 2001.

Vyas, Bharti with Haggard, Claire, *Beauty Wisdom: The Secret of Looking and Feeling Fabulous*, Thorsons, 1997.

Wildwood, Chrissie, *The Bloomsbury Encyclopedia of Aromatherapy*, Bloomsbury, 1996.

Wilson, Paul, *Calm at Work*, Penguin Books, 1998.

Address Book

UK

BODYWORK

Aromatherapy Organisations Council
PO Box 19834
London SE25 6WF
Tel: 020 8251 7912
www.aromatherapy-uk.org

British Acupuncture Council
Park House
206–208 Latimer Road
London W10 6RE
Tel: 020 8735 0400
www.acupuncture.org.uk

British Massage Therapy Council
17 Rymers Lane
Oxford OX4 3JU
Tel: 01865 774123
www.bmtc.co.uk

Society of Teachers of the
Alexander Technique
129 Camden Mews
London NW1 9AH
Tel: 020 7284 3338
www.stat.org.uk

EXERCISE

Body Control Pilates Association
14 Neal's Yard
London WC2H 9DP
Tel: 020 7379 3734
www.bodycontrol.co.uk

British Wheel of Yoga
1 Hamilton Place
Boston Road
Sleaford
Lincolnshire NG34 7ES
Tel: 01529 306851
www.bwy.org.uk

The Pilates Foundation
80 Camden Road
London E17 7NF
Tel: 07071 781859
www.pilatesfoundation.com

T'ai Chi Union of Great Britain
94 Felsham Road
London SW15 1DQ
Tel: 020 8780 1063
E-mail: comptonph@aol.com

Tse Qi Gong Centre
Tel: 01619 294485
www.bodytao.co.uk

HOLISTIC MEDICINE

Council for Complementary
and Alternative Medicine
Park House
206–208 Latimer Road
London W10 6RE
Tel: 020 8735 0400
www.acupuncture.org.uk

General Council and Register
of Naturopaths
2 Goswell Road
Street, Somerset BA16 0JG
Tel: 01458 840072
www.naturopathy.org.uk

National Institute of Medical Herbalists
56 Longbrooke Street
Exeter EX4 8HA
Tel: 01392 426022
www.btinternet.com/~nimh

The Society of Homeopaths
2 Arizan Road
Northampton NN1 4HU
Tel: 01604 621400
www.homeopathy-soh.org

MIND/BODY THERAPIES

British Association for Counselling
and Psychotherapy
1 Regent Place
Rugby
Warwickshire CV21 3PJ
Tel: 08704 435252
www.bac.co.uk

British Autogenic Society
Royal London Homoeopathic Hospital
Great Ormond Street
London WC1N 3HR
Tel: 020 7713 6336
www.autogenic-therapy.org.uk

MIND/National Association
for Mental Health
Granta House
15–19 Broadway
London E15 4BQ
Tel: 020 8519 2122/020 8522 1725
Information line operates from 9.15 am to
4.45 pm Monday, Wednesday, Thursday,
Friday and from 2 pm to 4.45 pm Tuesday.
www.mind.org.uk

No Panic
93 Brands Farm Way
Telford
Shropshire TF3 2JQ
Tel: 01952 590005 (office)
Tel: 01952 590545 (help line)
www.no-panic.co.uk

Transcendental Meditation
Freepost
London SW1P 4YY
Tel: 08705 143733
wwww.t-m.org.uk

NUTRITION
The Institute for Optimum Nutrition
13 Blades Court
Deodar Road
London SW15 2NU
Tel: 020 8877 9993
www.ion.ac.uk

The Nutri Centre
The Hale Clinic
7 Park Crescent
London W1N 3HE
Tel: 020 7436 5122
www.nutricentre.com

Society for the Promotion
of Nutritional Therapy
BCM Box SPNT
London WC1N 3XX
www.nutritionaltherapy.co.uk

RETREATS
The Retreat Company
The Manor House
Kings Norton
Leicestershire LE7 9BA
Tel: 01162 599211
www.retreat-co.co.uk

USA

Alexander Technique Center
Email: info@alexandercenter.com
www.alexandercenter.com

American Association of Acupuncture
and Oriental Medicine
4101 Lake Boone Trail Suite 201
Raleigh, NC 27607
Tel: 919 787 5181
www.holisticmedicine.com

American Chiropractic Association
1701 Clarendon Blvd
Arlington, VA 22209
Tel: 703 276 8800
www.acatoday.com

American Herbalist Guild
1931 Gaddis Road
Canton GA 30115
Tel: 770 751 6021
www.americanherbalistguild.com

Body/Mind Restoration Retreats
56 Lieb Road
Spencer, NY 14883
Tel: 607 272 0694
www.bodymindretreats.com

International Association
of Yoga Therapists
2400A County Center Drive
Santa Rosa, CA 95403
Tel: 707 566 9000
www.iayt.org

The National Association
for Holistic Aromatherapy
4509 Interlake Avenue North
Seattle, WA 98103-6773
Tel: 206 547 2164
www.naha.org

National Certification Board for
Therapeutic Massage and Bodywork
8201 Greensboro Drive, Suite 300
McLean, VA 22102
Tel: 800 296 0664
www.ncbtmb.com

Nutritional Center for Homeopathy
801 North Fairfax Street, Suite 306
Alexandria, VA 22314
Tel: 703 548 7790
www.homeopathy.org

CANADA

Acupuncture Canada
107 Leitch Drive
Grimsby, Ontario L3M 2T9
Tel: 905 563 8930
www.acupuncture.ca

The Canadian Herb Society
5251 Oak Street
Vancouver, British Columbia V6M 4H1
www.herbsociety.ca

Tzu Chi Institute for
Complementary Medicine
767 West 12th Avenue
Vancouver, British Columbia V5Z 1M9
Tel: 604 875 4769
www.tzu-chi.ba.ca

AUSTRALIA

Association of Traditional Health
Practitioners Incorporated
PO Box 346
Elizabeth, South Australia 5112
Tel: 08 8284 2324
www.traditionalmedicine.net.au

Australian Homeopathic Association
PO Box 396
Drummoyne, New South Wales 2047
Tel: 02 9719 2793

National Herbalist Association of Australia
33 Reserve Street
Annandale, New South West 2038
Tel: 02 9560 7077
www.nhaa.org.au

Index

Acknowledgements

Picture Credits

Hugh Arnold 90

Courtesy Bach Flower Remedies 103

© Carlton Books Ltd 90, 84, 119, 120 / Graham Atkins-
Hughes: 1, 8, 14, 35, 39, 41, 45, 54, 56tl, 58, 61, 85, 94,
96, 110 / Jason Bell: 86, 87, 88 / John Davis: 87 /
Catherine Gratwicke: 115 / Alistair Morrison: 34, 75 /
Lizzie Orme: 43, 91 / Photodisc Carlton: 32, 64 / Polly
Wreford: 28, 57tr, 57bl, 60, 62, 68tr, 92tl, 92bl, 93, 97,
114, 118

Sean Cook / Marie Claire Health and Beauty / IPC
Syndication 80

Flowerphotos 108

Foodpix 69

FPG 21, 26, 36, 42, 56tr, 69

Donna Francesca 82

Getty Images Stone 2–3, 4–5, 6, 11, 12, 16, 23br, 25, 31,
38, 44, 46br, 49, 56bl, 56br, 59br, 63, 66, 67c, 67bc,
68br, 71, 72, 76–77, 78bl, 78–79, 81, 98, 100, 101, 102,
105, 106, 107, 109, 112, 117

Imagebank 13, 18, 22, 23tr, 47, 50, 57tl, 57br, 65, 74, 123

PA photos 27

Pictor 10

Every effort has been made to acknowledge correctly and
contact the source and/or copyright holder of each picture
and Carlton Books Limited apologises for any unintentional
errors or omissions which will be corrected in future
editions of this book.

Author Acknowledgements

Without the support of the following people, this
book would have been much less of a pleasure to
write. Many thanks are due to my editors Venetia
Penfold and Zia Mattocks plus the rest of the
publishing team at Carlton, who have embodied
a rare combination of efficiency and good humour.
As always, my agent Teresa Chris has been a delight
to work with, providing moral and extremely
practical support in abundance. Drs Anand and
Anthea Anand also receive my warmest thanks for
taking time out of extremely busy schedules in order
to provide their constructive professional comments.

All of the titles in the Recommended Reading section
have been instrumental in opening my eyes to fresh
perspectives on stress, but the books listed by
Chrissie Wildwood, Bharti Vyas and Leslie Kenton
have been particular sources of inspiration within the
field of holistic approaches to health and beauty. All
my love goes to Denis, who is always there when
the going gets tough. Without his constant support,
life would never be the same. Last, but not least, my
cat Samantha must be mentioned as being the best
aid to stress management an author could have.